BODY POLLUTION

BODY POLLUTION

GARY NULL and STAFF

Edited by James Dawson

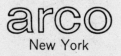

New York

Fourth Printing, 1977

Published by Arco Publishing Company, Inc.
219 Park Avenue South, New York, N.Y. 10003

Copyright © 1973 by Gary Null

Library of Congress Catalog Number 72–92307

ISBN 0–668–02904–8

Printed in U.S.A.

Contents

1.	Body Pollution: The Crisis in Our Health	1
2.	Fertilizers	17
3.	Hidden Disaster—Food Additives	27
4.	The Biggest Worry—Carcinogens	35
5.	Surrogate Nutrition—Synthetics and Substitutes	61
6.	Pollution by Cosmetics and Drugs	71
7.	Drugs	81
8.	Our Sad State of Health	95
9.	Emotional and Mental Illness	121
10.	Alcoholism	131
11.	Who Is Responsible?	143
12.	Taking Action	165
13.	Immediate Personal Action	173
14.	Improved Diet	187
15.	Know What You Are Buying: Handbook of Additives	195
	Bibliography	205
	Index	207

BODY
POLLUTION

Body Pollution: The Crisis in Our Health

You, like most Americans, probably buy your food in a supermarket or corner grocery store. Almost any food you buy—whether boxed, canned, plastic wrapped, or unpackaged—is doused, impregnated, or immersed in chemicals that color, preserve, or in some way enhance its looks, crispness, or flavor. All this is done at the expense of your health. Most of the chemicals used by food suppliers and processors harmfully affect your body. The small amounts you take in daily with your food remain in your system. Large doses of many of these chemicals can kill you.

Although additives used in processing food are harmful chemicals, the most poisonous substances in your daily diet are pesticides, or pest-killers, used as crop sprays. Residues or sprays are found in almost all kinds of foodstuffs, including milk and baby foods.

The small amounts of poisons you take into your body every day gradually harm the function of your tissues and organs. In other words, the chemicals added to your foods slowly *pollute* your body. Thus, body pollution is the destruction, weakening, or poisoning of the body or many of its parts by the continued intake of artificial chemical substances in food.

The seriousness of the problem of body pollution cannot be overemphasized. We all must eat, and very few of us can grow

1

and process our food. Almost everyone, then, must eat foods that contain harmful chemicals, whether he wants to or not. Every year in the United States more than 150 deaths are traced directly to crop sprays, and other deaths are attributable to chemical food additives.

Tragic as these deaths may be, even more serious is the slow body pollution of the whole population in daily doses.

The American Medical Association's Council on Pharmacy and Chemistry has said that it is not reasonable to expect that the human body can escape injury if it is exposed year after year to small amounts of poisons. The AMA adds that *"the resultant injury may be cumulative or delayed, or simulate a chronic disease of other origin, thereby making identification and statistical comparison difficult or impossible."* Thus, we have no direct way of knowing the extent to which our whole population is slowly being poisoned by harmful chemicals in its food. Truly, the problem of body pollution is a real health crisis.

Causes of Body Pollution: Sprays, Fertilizers, and Other Chemicals Used in Food Production

Harmful substances that are added to food during processing and preserving can be controlled—although they rarely are—but poisons added accidentally are, of course, beyond control. The main group of poisonous substances added in this manner are chemical pesticides in the form of crop sprays.

There are four main kinds of crop sprays: (1) insecticides, (2) fungicides, (3) miticides, and (4) herbicides.

The largest of these groups is insecticides, of which there are five types: chlorinated hydrocarbons, carbamates, organic phosphates, inorganics, and synergists. These will be discussed shortly.

The Case of DDT

In 1972, the well-known chlorinated hydrocarbon insecticide, DDT, was banned from general use in the United States. The case of DDT, its history, disastrous use, and final banning make up a good illustration of what can happen when shortsighted and thoughtless use is made of modern science.

The chemical compound dichloro-diphenyl-trichloroethane (DDT) was first synthesized by a German chemist in 1874, but did not come into use until World War Two. During that war, DDT seemed like an answer to a public health doctor's prayer. Because of DDT powder there was not a single outbreak of typhus fever or cholera among American troops, their prisoners, or the civilian populations of the territories in which the troops fought. The spraying of DDT on South Pacific islands nearly eradicated malaria-carrying mosquitoes. With such accomplishments to its credit, it is no wonder that DDT was used by crop growers to rid their crops of insects when the war was over. DDT knocked out insects by the billions, and its manufacture and use skyrocketed.

The desire of the growers to get a good insecticide is understandable. Dr. John L. George, associate curator of mammals at the New York Zoological Park, says in a pamphlet prepared for the Conservation Foundation of New York: "In this Age of Insects when perhaps 60 to 80 per cent of all forms of life are members of this one class, it is not surprising that man has willingly sought methods of control. . . . It is estimated that there is an 11 billion dollar yearly loss of food and fiber harvests in the U.S. traceable to insects, fungi, and other animal or plant pests."

It was not long, however, before many people realized that DDT was not the blessing it had at first seemed. Indeed, when it was first introduced in America DDT was known to be toxic to human beings and other animals. In 1950, barely five years after DDT was put on the market, Dr. Morton S. Biskind warned a committee from the House of Representatives: "The introduction for uncontrolled general use by the public of the insecticide 'DDT' . . . and the series of even more deadly substances that followed has no previous counterpart in history. Beyond question, no other substance known to man was ever developed so rapidly and spread so indiscriminately over so large a portion of the earth in so short a time. This is the more surprising as, at the time DDT was released for public use, a large amount of data was already available in the medical literature showing that this agent was extremely toxic for many different species of animals, that it was cumulatively stored in the body fat, and that it appeared in the milk." At this time a few cases of DDT poisoning in human beings were also being reported, but these observations were almost completely ignored or misinterpreted.

Dr. Biskind went on to explain that a large number of cases of "virus X" and "intestinal flu" are really incidents of DDT poisoning by foods in which there were larger-than-usual residues of DDT.

Residues: Allowable and Actual

William Longgood, Pulitzer Prize-winning reporter, writes that when DDT was first put on the market, the Food and Drug Administration recommended its use in barns and on cows. Within four years, data had accumulated showing that "even if DDT was used merely in the barns, with feeding troughs covered, and the cows outside while it was being applied, the poison would appear in the milk within 24 hours." This caused the FDA to withdraw its recommendation for the use of DDT in dairying. Then, for many years, "the FDA took the strong position that no pesticide residue whatsoever could be permitted in milk; this made it illegal for milk containing *any* DDT to pass from one state to another."

Manufacturers of DDT and other pesticides wanted the

FDA to set limits of pesticides that could be tolerated in various foods. The FDA stuck to its guns. In 1958, it refused to grant tolerances to two chemicals—malathion and methoxychlor—both considered less poisonous than DDT. The FDA said clearly that there could be no pesticide residues in milk in any degree whatsoever and therefore the tolerance levels of both the pesticides would remain zero.

Longgood goes on to point out that the FDA soon found that 62 per cent of the milk in a nationwide test contained DDT; so did 75 per cent of the butter and 50 per cent of the cheese. By 1968, the government realized the hopelessness of trying to keep DDT and other pesticides out of milk, so they set tolerances of these chemicals. They allowed 0.05 part per million (ppm) for whole milk and 1.25 ppm for milk fat.

Although any pesticide in milk is too much, the tolerances are rarely, if ever, adhered to. It is probably impossible to buy any milk through the ordinary commercial channels that meets the FDA's tolerances. Thus, none of us escapes pollution of our bodies by DDT.

This is a serious problem insofar as infants are concerned. Babies have been shown to be especially susceptible to pesticide poisoning. DDT collects in the fatty tissues of the body, and since most infants are fat, they store up proportionately more DDT than an adult. When a baby learns to walk, it uses up its reserve of fat, and the stored DDT is released into the bloodstream, where it can be found in high concentrations.

What Now?

In the summer of 1972, the use of DDT was banned for general use as an insecticide. This action was the result of a long struggle. On one side were pesticide manufacturers, many large crop growers, and less-than-honest or stupid bureaucrats. On the other side were members of health and conservation groups, many physicians, and honest, public spirited employees of the FDA and other government regulatory agencies. The battle took place in Congress too, with congressmen and senators struggling on both sides of the fight.

Now that the war to ban DDT has been won, can we rest assured that all danger from this spray chemical is gone? Not at all. As we have seen, DDT is a *cumulative* poison. Not only does it accumulate in the body, but it remains there for very long periods—just how long is not known. One government department measured the amounts of DDT in the body fat of two men who had worked with this insecticide. They had 91 and 291 ppm of DDT in their body fat. "Even after prolonged rest from their occupations," a report said, "the DDT levels in their fat were still 30 and 240 ppm."

The people of most of the world's industrialized nations have been exposed to DDT for more than two and one-half decades. They have been taking in daily doses of DDT in their foods for all those years. Three generations of infants have nursed on milk contaminated with DDT. No one knows how long it would take for our bodies to eliminate all of it if DDT were suddenly absent from our environment, if indeed we could ever get rid of it all.

However, the fact is that the end of the use of DDT as a chemical spray does not mean that it still cannot get into our food. This chemical is very stable—not easily decomposed or broken down—in soil. Test plots of soil powdered with DDT retained 80 per cent of the chemical seven years later. Many farmers have been spraying crop fields for as many as 26 years, each year's amount adding to the DDT already in the soil. No one knows how long it will take for the soil of these fields to rid itself of the insecticide. It has been shown that crops grown in DDT-contaminated soil absorb the chemical. Thus, we will be eating DDT for many years to come, even though it is now illegal and out of use.

Unfortunately, DDT is only one of a large number of pesticides that can pollute the bodies of human beings and other animals.

Other Pesticide Poisons

There are a large number of pesticides on the market, and that number increases every year as research laboratories continually turn out new pest-killers. To get a good idea of how big the pesticide problem is, it is worth seeing what the field of these chemicals looks like. Dr. John L. George of the New York Zoological Park, summarizes the characteristics of pesticides as follows:

"*Chlorinated Hydrocarbons.* These chemicals typically are characterized by: (1) slow knockdown of insects; (2) high kill of insects; (3) high residual effect—very stable. Most are contact poisons to insects, . . . but become stomach poisons to those animals ingesting the intoxicated insects [for example, birds and fish]."

Besides DDT, other members of the chlorinated hydrocarbons are *Aldrin;* BHC (also known as HCH), one form of which is called *Lindane; Chlordane;* DDD, also known as TDE or *Rhothane;* DDE; *Dieldrin; Endrin; Isodrin; Methoxychlor; Perthane; Q137;* and *Toxaphene.* Dr. George continues:

"*The Organic Phosphates.* These compounds are characterized by (1) high initial knockdown of insects; (2) high kill; (3) low residual effect, *i.e.,* fairly rapid breakdown; (4) great toxicity to higher vertebrates [including man] in many cases. For example, TEPP is approximately 250 times as toxic to laboratory rats as DDT. . . .

"Commonly used toxins in this group are: *Chlorthion, Demeton; Diazinon; Dipterex;* EPN; *Malathion; Parthion; Schradon;* TEPP (tetraethyl pyrophosphate), also known as *Bladan* and TEP.

"*Carbamates.* This group includes *Dimetan,* . . . *Propamat,* . . . and *Pyrolan.* . . ."

"*The Inorganic Insecticides.* This is an old-time group but it is still in use. Commonly used insecticides of this group are: *arsenic* compounds, mainly calcium and lead arsenates; *barium* compounds; *boron* compounds; *copper* compounds; *fluorine* compounds (*Cryolite* is sodium aluminofluoride); *mercury* compounds; *selenium* compounds; *sulfur* compounds; *thallium* compounds; *zinc* compounds; elemental *phosphorus;* elemental *sulfur.*

"*Synergists.* Compounds or insecticides used in combination with other toxins to increase killing power."

There are not quite as many fungicides, miticides, and herbicides as insecticides, but there are still a considerable number of them. What is important about these pesticides is that almost all of them have been found to be poisonous to some degree. Still more important is the fact that there has not been enough research to tell us how these chemicals act in the body. In 1960, a high FDA official disclosed that one-third of all processed dairy products sampled by his agency in the previous few months had been contaminated with pesticide residues. "We need much more research," he said, "to give us basic information about pesticides and what they will do."

The most poisonous pesticides have been in use in the U.S. for no more than 27 years. Chlorinated hydrocarbons, starting with DDT, have been on the market since 1945. Organic phosphates have been used since 1947. Systemic insecticides (those that enter the plant's tissues and are taken in by sucking insects) were introduced in 1950. Several other kinds of pesticides came later.

Scientists have estimated that a thorough investigation of the cancer-producing potential of any substance takes 25 years. Only a few of the modern pesticides have been in use that long, and no research on their cancer-producing or other poisonous properties was begun until at least two years after they were in use. Therefore, we do not have a solid basis for giving any pesticide a clean bill of health.

Dr. Robert N. Goodman, a plant pathologist, pointed out that although there may be important differences among plants, animals, insects, and microorganisms, their metabolism on the individual cell level is essentially the same. Therefore, an insect poison is generally an animal, plant or microorganism poison, too.

A serious concern about all pesticides is that they may do their damage in very small doses. In 1959, two scientists, William F. Durham and Homer R. Wolfe, made a study of the potential hazard of small quantities of pesticides eaten as residues in harvested produce. They said that they were not aware of any case of illness from pesticide residues on food where pesticide formulations were used according to direction. However, they pointed out that there were several cases of poisoning where pesticides were used improperly.

The scientists went on to say, "The primary toxicological problem associated with residues, however, is not the possibility of a single exposure producing illness, but rather the possible adverse effect on health of consumption of small amounts of these chemicals over a period of years."

The long-term effect of any poison need not come about because the poison is stored in the body. William Longgood points out that it is a basic fact of toxicology that the damage done by each dose of a continued dosage of poison may add to the previous damage. Each daily intake of a pesticide may do damage that adds to that of the previous day's intake until serious and permanent damage is done to the body.

Direct Deaths From Pesticides

One June day, a mother was giving her five-year-old son a bath. The weather was warm enough to leave the window open. A couple of elm trees in front of the house were being sprayed and some of the fumes blew into the bathroom. The mother and son choked and coughed for 15 minutes.

Eight months later, the little boy was admitted to a hospital because of a skin wound that would not heal. His condition was diagnosed as acute granulocytic leukemia, and by the following June he was dead. Eight months later, his mother was found to have the same disease, and she followed her son in death.

At 8:30 A.M. on a day in November, 1967, a child died in the Colombian town of Chiquinquirá. By midafternoon, more than 130 other persons, many of them children, had become violently ill and near death.

It was found that a pint of the pesticide *Parthion* had leaked into bags of flour in a truck that was transporting them from Bogotá. Bread baked from the flour had transferred the insecticide to the 130 townspeople.

A month earlier, 17 people in Tijuana, Mexico, had died from Parthion-contaminated flour in their bread.

Parthion has been responsible for thousands of illnesses and many deaths in other parts of the world. The *Nippon Times* of Japan, reported:

"A total of 2,194 farmers and their family members were affected by the agricultural drug 'Parthion' last year, bringing deaths to 307 and physical disorders to 1,887 others. . . .

"Some 1,747 persons were affected by the drug while they were spraying it, 191 poisoned by stepping into places where the drug had been sprayed, 237 committed suicide by taking it, eight were poisoned by mishandling it, etc.

"A child died after he played in a river near a place where the drug had been sprayed.

"Six persons died from eating vegetables and fruits sprayed with the drug."

In one year, the state of Washington had over 100 pesticide poisonings, two fatal. Most were due to Parthion, the others to Demeton and Phosdrin, all organic phosphates.

One of the most efficient methods of applying pesticides is spraying them from a low-flying airplane. A number of "crop dusting" pilots have died because of their continual proximity to these chemicals. One Nebraskan pilot crashed and dragged himself unharmed from the wreckage of his plane, crawling through a pool of Parthion which had leaked from his tanks. With his clothes soaked with the liquid pesticide, he walked one and a half miles to a camp. An hour later, the pilot experienced headache, stomach cramps, nausea, and blurred vision. He was taken to a hospital, where he died within hours.

A crop duster crashed outside of Belpre, Ohio, in 1968. By evening eleven people had to be hospitalized, and three of them, including the pilot, died. A nearby dairy farm lost most of its cattle and had to stop milking the survivors.

One farmer lost all his cattle and hogs within a few minutes after he sprayed them heavily with TEPP. The farmer said that the container the chemical came in was marked "TEPP—40 per cent," followed by a warning to wash with water if any of the pesticide spilled on the skin and to call a doctor if taken internally. There were no other instructions. The container also had pictures of farm animals, from which the farmer inferred that animals were to be sprayed directly.

Many children are killed by pesticides each year. These pitiful victims usually touch the chemical with their hands and then suck their fingers. Keeping farm and garden pesticides out of the reach of children cannot be emphasized too strongly.

Specific Effects of Pesticides

Research has pinpointed how some pesticides do their terrible body-polluting work. Dr. Kenneth P. DuBois, Professor of Pharmacology at the University of Chicago, found that pesticides interfere with the desired effects of medicines. The pesticides neutralize some medications and make others more toxic. For example, DDT cancels the effects of barbiturates.

Dr. DuBois found that even at the permissible levels set by

the FDA, the organic phosphate pesticides inhibit the functioning of cholinesterase, the body chemical that carries nerve impulses. These same pesticides also interfere with the working of enzymes that ordinarily remove toxic substances from the body.

Another researcher found that DDT and other chlorinated hydrocarbons can seriously affect human sex organs.

Some pesticides cause effects that mimic psychological disorders. Scientists at the University of Colorado Medical Center found that men exposed to pesticides over a long time have slow reaction times, poor memories, and may lose their vitality and become very irritable. Slowness of thinking was another symptom of exposure to the organophosphates.

A psychiatrist, Dr. Douglas Gordon Campbell, of the University of California Medical School, said in 1963 that when a physician takes a case history, he should ask the patient if he uses pesticide sprays in his home or garden or on his job. An affirmative answer may explain symptoms that otherwise seem to be caused by psychological difficulties.

Naturalists have known for some time that DDT causes birds to lay eggs with extremely thin shells and which never hatch. This effect has led to the near extinction of some species of birds, such as the golden eagle. Dr. William L. Heinrichs, of the University of Washington, found that DDT can interfere with reproduction in mammals. He believes that an increase in the number of ovarian cysts among young women may be the result of exposure to DDT.

Have Pesticides Done Their Work?

In addition to the direct and indirect poisonings by modern pesticides, there is evidence that these chemicals have not been successful in their pest-killing mission. In the *1952 Yearbook of Agriculture*, former Secretary of Agriculture Charles F. Brannan wrote, "We have more insect pests although we have better insecticides and better ways to fight them."

Scientists have found that simple organisms such as insects, mites, and fungi can build up a resistance to pesticides and pass the resistance on to subsequent generations. One result of this genetic immunity to pesticides has been that man develops new, more powerful chemicals and escalates the war on pests. Despite these efforts, the pests have been winning.

When DDT was first used, it killed malaria-carrying mosquitoes by the billions. Public health officials predicted the day when the miracle pesticide would wipe out malaria all over the world. However, it was not long before they found that some mosquitoes had developed an immunity to DDT. Public health officials are now extremely worried by the resurgence of malaria where it was believed to have been wiped out. The new breed of malaria-carrying mosquitoes seem to be immune to most sprays. Among the few pesticides that are still effective are the organophosphates, but, as we have seen, these are most poisonous to man.

Insecticides usually do not discriminate among insects, and kill the useful along with the harmful. Bees are killed as efficiently as borers. When birds eat poisoned insects and die, those insects they fed upon then multiply out of control.

Insecticides and other pesticides collect in the soil, which is made up of small particles of rock and decaying organic matter, and huge numbers of living things, from earthworms to actinomycetes to bacteria, most of which are very beneficial in keeping soil fertile. If these living things are killed by pesticides, the soil deteriorates.

Longgood writes that the primary drawback of all pesticides, in addition to their poisonous effect on man, is that they upset the balance of nature. For example, if a large number of insects hatch in a certain year, they provide more food for birds, which then increase in numbers. The increased number of birds eats more insects, lowering the insect population. Then, with less to eat, the bird population is reduced, and the former balance of insects and birds is re-established. As we have seen, if birds are killed by eating pesticide-impregnated insects, the insects will then be able to multiply out of control.

The development of miticides resulted in an upset of the balance of nature. Mites were not considered to be important pests because their numbers were kept in control by insect enemies. When insecticides killed off these insects, mites became important pests. Then it was necessary to develop miticides to kill the mites.

Harmless Pesticides

There are a number of pesticides that have been known for many years, some for centuries. They come from various plants and are called *botanicals*. Most are safe to warm-blooded animals, but a few, among them nicotine, are very poisonous. A very effective and harmless insecticide is pyrethrum, which is obtained from two species of chrysanthemums. Another natural insecticide is rotenone, which comes from the root of the derris plant.

A promising way of killing insect pests without harming man or other animals is using atomic radiation to sterilize male insects of the species under attack. The sterile males are released at breeding times, and the females with which they breed lay sterile eggs that never hatch. This method has been used to wipe out infestations of screw worm flies in several parts of the United States, and has also been effective against the Mediterranean fruit fly. No harmful effects from this method have been reported.

Natural Resistance to Pests

Probably the best way to combat crop pests is to breed species of grain, fruits, and vegetables that have a natural resistance to insects, mites, and fungi. This can be done, and there are many such species in existence. With enough work and with the money spent for chemical pesticide research, there is no doubt that many more resistant kinds of crops could be bred.

The Future of Pesticides

Although the banning of DDT, Dieldrin and a few other pesticides is a step in the right direction, it is only a beginning. New pesticides replace those banned and the harmful, polluting effects of pesticides on the human body continue. People who worry about these effects must join those who successfully brought about the banning of a few pesticides and continue the fight in and out of government.

New legislation is needed, a Federal Environment Pesticide Control Act, under which the Administrator of the Environmental Protection Agency would be required to classify pesticides as "for general use," "for restricted use," or "for use by permit only." This would keep the most dangerous pesticides out of inexperienced hands.

But no legislative act can eliminate the dangers of pesticide use. There are not nearly enough inspectors to see that the law is obeyed, and no law can do anything about the cumulative effects of even those pesticides that are considered "safe." The way things stand, the pollution of our bodies by pesticides seems destined to go on for some time into the future.

Fertilizers

For thousands of years, farmers fertilized their crops with the natural nutrients found in animal wastes—manure and dung—and in the rotting vegetable matter known as compost. Then, in the early nineteenth century, a German chemist, Justus von Liebig, performed a brilliant series of experiments through which he discovered the chemical substances plants need for growth. He concluded that if man provided these substances, plants would obtain from them all the nutrients they needed. This was the beginning of chemical fertilization of the soil.

To determine the chemical elements needed by vegetation, von Liebig burned plants, chemically analyzed the substances he found in the ashes, and concluded that soil was merely a mixture of those substances. As sound as this method may appear, it ignored the fact that soil is more than its mineral content. We now know that it is the organic content of soil that is necessary for the growth of healthy plants. This organic content is called *humus*. It is made up of decaying dead matter as well as numberless small living organisms.

Von Liebig failed to see soil as a living component in the overall scheme of nature. Being a laboratory chemist, he did not understand that the myriad of living things in soil—from moles, mice, and shrews to earthworms and microorganisms—is an essential, indispensable, life-supporting part of soil.

America's Crime Against Its Soil

Poor soil management has robbed our land of *half its topsoil* in 350 years. The seriousness of this loss becomes apparent when we consider that it takes 500 to 1,000 years to replace a single inch of topsoil. We have lost, in 350 years, somewhere between three and six thousand years of nature's work in creating fertile topsoil.

The greater part of our loss of topsoil was due to water erosion caused by the poor farming practices of early settlers and pioneers. Most of these farmers did not know how to conserve soil and they did not bother to learn because land was free or very cheap. "Get what crops you can out of the land, and when it is ruined, move on," was their credo. Today, most farmers, aware of the damage their forefathers did, are quite successful at combatting destruction of soil by erosion. (Now it is the builders of suburbs and roads that are destroying the soil through erosion.) How tragic, then, that the modern farmer has found a new way to destroy soil—by means of chemical fertilization.

We have already mentioned the failure of chemical farming to regard soil and plant growth in terms of whole systems. It is this one-sided thinking that is responsible for tremendous ecological imbalances today. Sir Albert Howard, a pioneer and moving force in organic farming, referred to this thinking as "fragmentation"—a way of regarding soil in its mineral, or chemical, aspect only. Fertilization of soil is only one part of the growing process, and it cannot function independently of the other parts. Organic farmers' main objection to chemical farming is its blindness to the life cycle in soil.

The majority of farmers in the United States depend entirely on chemical fertilization. More than seven million tons of high-nitrogen fertilizers are sold yearly in this country. Most of today's farmers do not know any other way to fertilize their crops. They have no clear idea of the complex natural relationships between the properties of soil and the organic matter that should be present in it, and make no effort to see that organic matter is part of their soil.

The internal combustion engine replaced the horse as a source of power and a means of transportation on farms. Today, the produce farmer buys meat from the butcher and milk from a store or dairy farm, instead of keeping cattle and pigs. He has therefore lost the cheap, easily available source of animal wastes—horse manure and cattle dung—that his forefathers had. This is an unfortunate loss; soil dressed with animal wastes produces crops that are more nourishing than those grown in chemically fertilized soil. Also, the substitution of chemical fertilizers for natural ones leads to soil deterioration. As this process goes on, crops steadily lose their nutritional vigor, and food that is losing its nutritiousness leads to deterioration in the health of the entire population.

Death of the Living Soil

Chemical fertilizers bring about unnatural changes in the make-up of soil that destroy or seriously disturb the living things that benefit the soil. The presence of these organisms serves as a barometer of soil fertility. If they cannot survive in the soil, it is a sign that the soil will not bear crops worth eating. The work of earthworms and microorganisms ordinarily can restore depleted soil, but not as long as the damage is being continued by chemical poisoning. For example, superphosphate fertilizers tend to create acid conditions within soil which kill earthworms. In Australia, nine-foot-long earthworms originally present in vast numbers were completely exterminated by this type of fertilizer.

This destruction of living things in soil is due to the fact that fertilizer ingredients are so readily water soluble. In nature, easily soluble plant food elements rarely occur. For example, humus harbors plant nutrients that dissolve in water very slowly, feeding plants at a rate which precludes the possibility of poisoning them and their living benefactors in the soil.

Soil that cannot support life within its own structure will not be able to fulfill the vital nutritional needs of human beings. On the other hand, the application of organic matter, fully or partially composted into humus, will improve the soil sufficiently for the living soil benefactors to exist in it. Withholding organic fertilizer from depleted soil make its revitalization impossible.

The subtle and gradual poisoning of the land was completely overlooked by most farmers in their instant and unquestioning acceptance of chemical farming. It took a few years before the detrimental effects became evident, but by that time the fertilizer industry had become so large that there was no stopping its crushing wheel of "progress."

Chemical destruction of soil is truly insidious—but it is no longer a secret. Yet it continues! The popularity of chemical crop growing is a disheartening testimony to man's vain attempts to outdo nature. On the other hand, organic gardening, working with natural materials which are the core of soil structure, is a hopeful symbol of the intelligent and fruitful manner in which man and nature can cooperate.

The Proper Use of Chemical Fertilizers

Many fertilizers which chemists construct include compounds so long-lasting that they eventually penetrate into the subsoil and disrupt the natural and desirable chemical and biological changes that take place there.

Organic materials act as buffers against over-powerful action by chemical fertilizers, so it is the chemical-using farmer who most needs organic materials in his soil. Sadly, these farmers are the ones who refuse organic buffering most vigorously.

Good farmers use chemical fertilizers only as supplements. They improve and strengthen the soil through organic methods and use caution when making supplements of the chemical fertilizers without serious soil and crop damage. Although most organic farmers would insist that this is certainly not proper, it *has* proved to be a sane and proper way of using chemical fertilizers.

Trace Elements

Fertilization of soil requires more than nitrogen, phosphorus, and potassium, the main ingredients of chemical fertilizers. Another group of elements, called trace elements, is needed. Although they make up only one per cent of a plant's needs, trace elements are very important for healthy and vigorous development of vegetation. Also, it has been found that many human diseases are the result of a diet deficient in trace elements, which can be easily obtained from foods grown in organically rich soil.

Chemical fertilizer manufacturers did not overlook the discovery of trace elements. Once they learned of it, they put trace elements into their products, calling them such things as "power boosters." Fertilizers containing trace elements must be used with the same restraint as any kind of chemical fertilizer. Careless use of these elements is detrimental to soil, the animals that live in it, and the plants that grow in it.

Improving the Soil's Sponge Structure

On any plot of extremely depleted soil, the most urgent need is the replacement of a healthy sponge structure. Such improvement requires the addition of organic materials. For example, the addition of chemical fertilizers to a sandy soil, not bound together by organic material, is almost futile because the applied plant food ingredients will trickle straight through. In the case of soil lacking a spongy structure because it is tightly packed clay, fertilizing substances will not be able to penetrate the soil at all. For these reasons, soil which has lost its spongy quality is hopelessly infertile. Hopeless, that is, unless the gardener or farmer works to re-establish a new sponge structure. He will never achieve this through the use of chemical fertilizers alone. He must use organic methods.

Pesticides and Fertilizers

There is a direct relationship between abuse of soil and the damage done by pesticides. Dr. Donald Lewis Mader of the University of Wisconsin has found that more DDT accumulates in soil which has lost its humus than in soil with a healthy, spongy structure. In other words, the more humus in soil, the less accumulation of pesticide poisons. Dr. Mader also found that the addition of chemical fertilizers increased the toxicity of pesticides in the soil.

Chemical Fertilizers and Nutrition

As we have seen, crops grown in soil overfertilized by chemicals are usually lacking in nutritive values. One experiment that proved this fact was done with hay at the University of West Virginia. Drs. Lana Bailey and Gary Kelley produced almost twice as much hay on fields given a chemical nitrogenous fertilizer as they did on unfertilized fields. The figures were 3,200 pounds of hay to a fertilized acre, compared to 1,700 to an unfertilized acre. However, when fed to rabbits, a pound of the nitrogen-fertilized hay produced less rabbit meat than a pound of the unfertilized hay. The nitrogen had forced the soil to produce more hay, but the hay, pound for pound, lacked the nutritive value of the hay grown naturally.

The well-known environmentalist, Dr. Barry Commoner, has pointed out that nitrogenous chemical fertilizers dissolved in rain water make their way to lakes and rivers, where they provide nourishment for water plants and cause them to grow

Hidden Disaster—
Food Additives

To remain healthy, your body must wage a daily struggle against not only the poisons that enter your food from pesticides and fertilizers, but also from the chemicals that are added to your food to make it look nicer, preserve it longer on food markets' shelves, make it crisper or softer, or change it in many other ways.

When you shop in a supermarket or your neighborhood grocery store, you have no choice but to buy food that contains scores of additives. Mrs. Ione Dennis Starkey, a consumer-minded housewife, testifying before a congressional hearing on coloring additives, said, "The shopper, really informed and looking for plain food with nothing added or taken away, is like Diogenes with a lantern unable to find an honest man."

You are not ordinarily aware of the presence of the additives in your food. Some well-informed persons can tell by taste and looks that certain additives are in a food, but most are invisible and do not make their presence known to any of your senses. There are thousands of additives approved by government authorities for use by producers and packers. A large proportion of these additives are made up of chemicals harmful to your health. Most of the rest are of no value to you as a consumer. Former Food and Drug Administration (FDA) Commissioner Dr. James L. Goddard told the Food Protection Committee of the National Academy of Science's National Research Council,

"In a number of cases the additives have only an economic benefit to the food producers and no benefit at all to the person who eats the final product."

Why Food Additives?

Additives are put into food for a number of reasons. Some are used as:

Antispoilants. These chemicals almost entirely prevent or greatly slow down the reproduction of bacteria, which is the cause of food spoilage. Foods to which antispoilants are added will keep for a long time—perhaps months—on a grocers' shelves. Many foods that previously spoiled overnight if not refrigerated, now can be kept on cupboard shelves for days without spoiling. In a refrigerator, these antispoilant-treated foods will last for very long times.

Flavorings. There are more than 2,000 flavoring additives, more than any other kind. About 500 flavors come from nature, the rest are synthetic.

Colors. These are dyes that make foods look tempting. For instance, pale yellow, green, or mottled oranges are dyed a rich orange color. Today, all oranges look good. Some foods have natural colors that fade after storage or during processing. Artificial coloring matter restores these foods to their original color, making them look fresh. For example, sodium nitrite gives processed meats a healthy-looking red hue.

Processing Aids. These additives make processing easier. There are antifoaming agents that prevent or minimize the formation of foam in large vats of liquid foods, such as soups. The fermentation of wine produces foam, which can make transport and bottling difficult, so the wine industry uses silicones to control foaming.

Moisture Controls. These additives increase or decrease the amount of moisture in foods. Glycerine, which absorbs moisture from the air, is put into marshmallows to keep them moist and soft. Table salt may be kept from caking because of moisture in the air, by adding calcium silicate.

Acid-Alkaline Controls. Certain foods must have just the right amount of acidity or alkalinity. A number of acids, alkalis, and salts may be added to foods to keep them properly acid or alkaline. Salts of citric acid are added to jellies and phosphoric acid is added to soft drinks for this purpose.

Agents That Improve Functional Properties. These additives are thickeners and firming, jelling, and maturing agents. Some form emulsions and suspensions. Watery canned tomatoes may be thickened by the addition of certain calcium salts.

Physiologic Activity Agents. These are added to fresh fruits and vegetables to hasten ripening or to slow down growth activities after harvesting. For example, ethylene glycol is a gas used to speed up the ripening of bananas, and maleic hydride prevents stored potatoes from sprouting.

Nutrition Supplements. Foods are "enriched" with vitamins, minerals, and amino acids. The wrapper of almost any loaf of bread will list a number of nutrition supplements such as thiamine, riboflavin, iron, and ascorbic acid as enrichers of the bread.

The Harm Food Additive Chemicals Can Do

Some additives cause changes in the food, destroying vitamins, changing the natural chemical structure of the food materials, or reacting with the food materials to actually produce poisons.

Other additives leave the food unchanged, but affect your body. These may act slowly, causing no immediate illness that is easily detectable. However, there may be harmful effects such as enlargement of vital organs that have been struggling to fight off the poisons. Also, there are microscopic changes to bodily organs that can be detected only by a pathologist.

Many food additives prevent vitamins and enzymes from

fulfilling their natural roles in the body's normal functioning. The results of this interference are vitamin deficiencies and malfunctioning of bodily processes due to lack of necessary enzymes. Physicians recognize vitamin and enzyme deficiency in symptoms such as constipation, loss of appetite, weakness, headache, disturbed sleep, inability to concentrate, unusual irritability, stomach gas, and burning tongue. Worse yet, long-continued vitamin and enzyme deficiency can result in serious illness.

Catalase is an enzyme found in almost all living cells of plants and animals, including human beings. It is important in controlling cell respiration—the taking in of oxygen and the excretion of carbon dioxide by cells. Catalase sets up a barrier to virus infections, certain poisonous substances, and to certain cancer-producing agents. Some food additives destroy catalase. Without catalase, a cell is open not only to virus invasion and toxins, but may develop abnormalities that result in cancer.

Dr. R. A. Holman, writing in *The Journal of the Soil Association* (1960), said, "It is obvious that if the fundamental biological mechanism is interfered with for a long enough time by physical and chemical agents present in our environment, whether in food, drink, drugs, or in the air we breathe, then we shall see in races so exposed a progressive increase in the incidence of cancer. By contrast, in those primitive communities where such agents are not used or encouraged, the incidence will remain at a very low level. In my opinion most of the chemicals added to food and drink for preservation or coloring could and should be abolished."

The Government Stands Aside

Almost everyone has seen on food containers such phrases as "certified colors and flavors," or on meat, "U.S. Government Inspected." Such information gives most Americans the feeling that the government would not allow any harmful substances ever to have official approval for use in foods. This is a false sense of assurance. Actually, there have been (and still are) food additives known to be harmful which have had government approval. Some substances approved by the Food and Drug Administration at one time were later banned because their harmfulness was discovered by other government agencies or nongovernment investigators. Some of these additives are Red Dye No. 1 and Butter Yellow, two coal tar dyes; safrole, a synthetic flavoring; and cyclamate, a synthetic sweetener.

The fact that a substance has had government approval for a long time does not mean that it has been safe during all that time. Dulcin, an artificial sweetener, was used for 50 years with government approval before being banned. Agene, a very widely used flour bleach, had 30 government-okayed years to do its harm, and the synthetic flavoring, coumarin, was used for 70 years before it was forbidden.

Former FDA Commissioner George P. Larrick wrote in the *Food, Drug, and Cosmetic Law Journal* (June 1957), "We have had some very narrow escapes because of the use of additives that had no place in food. It is inconceivable that this country should continue to expose itself indefinitely to the risks inherent in the present scheme of food control." Unfortunately, it seems that tragedy must strike again and again before action is taken to get rid of harmful food additives. Lithium chloride, a salt substitute, caused several deaths before its poisonous properties were recognized and it was banned. A salt of the element cobalt was approved as a foaming agent in beer by both the FDA and the Canadian Food and Drug Directorate. After nearly 100 heavy beer drinkers died of heart attacks, the foaming agent was found to be the cause and was forbidden by both governments.

Unsafe, but Still Permitted

Under existing procedures, it is possible for an additive to be known as harmful and yet not be banned entirely from use. A case in point concerns NDGA (nordihydroguairetic acid) which was used in shortening, soft drinks, cake mixes, and meats for the purpose of slowing down oxidation. The FDA had NDGA on its GRAS (Generally Recognized As Safe) list. The UN's Joint FAO/WHO Expert Food Additives Committee reviewed available scientific data on NDGA, and found no cause for alarm. The Canadian Food and Drug Directorate scrutinized the UN committee's report and concluded that it was inadequate, and carried out its own investigation of NDGA. It found that, in levels as low as 0.5 per cent, NDGA produced in rats depressed growth, hemorrhaging, lesions in lymph nodes, and enlarged kidneys with cysts. The FDD's Director General, R. A. Chapman, told Canadian food processors, on September 20, 1967, that NGDA "may result in hazards to health" and he recommended banning the additive from foods.

In the United States, the FDA realized that it could no longer keep NDGA on its Generally Recognized As Safe list, even though it had just extended the clearance of NDGA (and other oxidants) to be used in dry sausage.

Two months after the announcement of the Canadian ban on NDGA, the Food and Drug Administration said that it had conducted an investigation that had "complemented the Canadian studies." A short time afterward the FDA had to admit that it had not engaged in any study of its own. It said it would take action against NDGA because it had a "lack of sufficient toxicological data." One wonders what data the FDA used when approving the additive for its GRAS list in the first place.

In November 1967, the FDA announced that it proposed to remove NDGA from the GRAS list. Three large manufacturers protested, but the FDA said that their arguments provided "no substantive evidence to alter the proposed course of action." The following April, NDGA was removed from GRAS, but it was reclassified as a food additive "for which a food additive regulation is necessary to permit its use." This means that

NDGA is not banned outright in the United States, as it was in Canada, but is merely off the GRAS list. Following the FDA's action, the U.S. Department of Agriculture banned NDGA in most meat products. Then, the Agriculture Department's Consumer and Marketing Service said that NDGA is safe for rendered fat products such as lard and shortening. If, as the FDA maintained, there is a "lack of sufficient toxicological data," how can NDGA be considered safe in any food product whatsoever?

Synergism–The Dangerous Combinations

The large number of food additives taken into your body at every meal poses more of a threat than is posed by each individual additive. The additives may form combinations that result in entirely new chemical substances. This is known as synergism. It is virtually impossible to tell what additives will combine, nor is it possible to know what substances are formed by the chemical reactions due to the combinations. In an average dinner meal, a hundred additives may be ingested. These can form literally millions of combinations. Fortunately, most combinations will not react, but enough will so that a real danger exists. The medical profession is beginning to realize that many cases of acute indigestion, vomiting, and sudden headaches are not due to spoiled food, as seems apparent, but are the result of toxins formed in the body by unknown combinations of food additives. Dr. Irving Selikoff, professor of environmental medicine at the Mt. Sinai School of Medicine, said in a broadcast, "We may eventually see diseases that we don't even begin to understand at this time. Also, the sum total of these various low-level contaminants—each in itself not very important—may be to generally shorten life."

Toxicologists have found that the toxicity of one chemical in a food additive may be strengthened greatly by interacting with another chemical additive present in the body at the same time.

The Biggest Worry— Carcinogens

Of all the diseases that can be caused by food additives, the most dreaded is, of course, cancer. As far back as the early 1960's, Dr. W. C. Heuper, a recognized cancer expert, classified more than a dozen categories of food chemicals as carcinogens—cancer producing agents. He made his classification "according to the widely accepted definition that carcinogens are agents which when applied under certain conditions to man or animals elicit the subsequent development of cancers which would not have appeared otherwise."

Some of the additives on Dr. Heuper's list are:

Certain food dyes. Among these are Yellow AB and Yellow OB, which are used to color butter, margarine, and some baked goods.

Hormones used for hastening the growth of livestock and poultry. One of these, diethylstilbestrol (DES), was banned in 1972 from use in cattle and poultry feed, because its cancer-producing action had been clearly established. Unfortunately, the ban did not include the placing of DES pellets under the skin of the ears of beef cattle.

Wrapping and coating materials composed of polymerized carbon and silicon compounds. These include several of the "see through" types of wrappings.

Paraffins and mineral oils, if insufficiently refined and employed for the coating of foods such as cheeses and fruits and the coating of paper and cardboard food containers.

Polycyclic aromatic compounds found in soot that adheres to smoked goods.

Synthetic mucilages, such as carboxymethyl cellulose, which are used as thickeners and stabilizers in processed cheese, ice cream, salad dressing, chocolate milk, pressure-dispensed whipped cream, sherbets, and other frozen products; also in nonfattening canned fruit syrups.

Flavoring agents. Lemon oil has been recently noted as a carcinogen. Many other flavoring substances which are derived from coal tar are under surveillance as possible carcinogens.

Surfactants. Antifoaming agents, dispersants, and emulsifiers may enter into synergistic relationships with known "weak carcinogens," making it possible for the cancer-producing substances to penetrate tissues that would not otherwise be reached.

Dr. Heuper points out that very many suspected carcinogens have not been subjected to adequate testing, some of which takes a long time—two or three decades. Known carcinogens are allowed in foods on the grounds that they are present in amounts so small as to do no harm. Apologists for these carcinogens point to the fact that their cancer-producing properties are known only from massive doses given to laboratory animals. But, the argument continues, when very much smaller amounts of the carcinogens are ingested by the human animal, which is so much larger than a laboratory mouse or rabbit, the action of the carcinogen can be ignored. The weak point of this argument is that we do not know whether small doses of a carcinogen, ingested over a period of years, will build up to cancer-producing strength. Dr. Heuper thinks that there is a real chance that they will.

Bread—Tasteless Cotton in a Wrapper

Anyone who has ever tasted homemade bread or bread sold in a small neighborhood bakery or a health food store must be disgusted by the bread sold in supermarkets and grocery stores. Former FDA Commissioner Paul Dunbar described the modern loaf of white bread as "cotton fluff wrapped up in a skin." The 1965–66 *Consumer Bulletin Annual* called the bread "presliced absorbent cotton." A columnist writing in the *Daily Mail* (England) said, "Our bread is sliced, wrapped, steamed, and whitened to duplicate the consistency of old newspapers . . . [it has an] unforgettable aroma of nothingness." What happened to store-bought bread?

Until about a century ago, wheat was ground between mill stone discs, where its whole grain was reduced to fine particles by the milling operation. Just about a century ago, the steel rolling mill was introduced, which crushed rather than ground the wheat grain. The bran and the healthful wheat germ were separated from the rest of the grain. When the flour was sifted, bran and wheat germ were left on the screens to be sold separately. The rest of the wheat grain—the starchy part—could be kept for long periods or shipped long distances without spoiling because it lacked the oily wheat germ. Also, lacking the brown coat—the bran—the flour was white and could be baked into white bread. For centuries, white bread has been associated with social distinction, while brown bread (the "black bread" of peasants) has been considered a mark of the lower social classes. Prior to the steel rolling mill, millers and bakers had lightened the color of their flour by adding lighteners such as powdered chalk. The new method of milling yielded cheap light-colored flour that could make white bread available to everyone.

It was soon found that steel-roller milled flour was lacking in many nutrients. Good-quality proteins, such as lysine and tryptophan, are removed. Unsaturated fatty acids and vitamin E are excluded from the flour along with the wheat germ.

Two researchers, Drs. Tom and Eloise McHenry, at the College of Agriculture of the University of California, found that valuable minerals were removed from the wheat in approximately the following percentages: manganese (98%), iron (80%), magnesium (75%), phosphorus (70%), copper (65%), calcium (50%), and potassium (50%). The same researchers found that the vitamin loss was approximately: thiamin (80%), niacin (75%), riboflavin (65%), pantothenic acid (50%), and pyridoxine (50%). In addition to the foregoing minerals and vitamins, several other food elements are removed by modern milling methods.

More than half a century ago, a miller decided that the light-colored flour resulting from steel-roller milling was not white enough. He discovered that flour could be further whitened by bleaching with chemicals. The most widely used bleach was agene (nitrogen trichloride). As far back as 1927, the British Ministry of Health, acting on the basis of laboratory experiments, recommended that agene be banned in food processing. Nothing was done about it. In the United States, dogs were observed to suffer from running fits that ended in epileptic-like seizures. In 1946, a British physician, Sir Edward Mellanby, proved that the fits were due to agene in bread. Tests in the United States agreed with Mellanby's conclusions. Finally, in 1949, agene was banned as a food bleach in the United States, but, despite its known danger, agene was not outlawed in Britain until 1956.

Agene was replaced by chlorine dioxide, a bleach that destroys any vitamin E that may remain in flour after the milling process. A 1961 article in the *British Medical Journal* said that even if no trace of chlorine dioxide remains in flour, the bleached product may contain toxic substances and have its nutritional value greatly impaired.

After milling out minerals and vitamins and then bleaching the remains, the modern "miller" sends the almost nutritionless flour to the baker. To bake a loaf of bread with whole milk, eggs, and butter is far too expensive for today's giant baking corporations which are in cutthroat competition for the consumers' dollars. So the baker puts into his nutritionless dough a minimum amount of powdered skim milk and powdered eggs and lardlike fat. He can then say on the wrapper that his bread contains wholesome milk, eggs, and shortening.

Unfortunately, there is an almost universal belief among food shoppers that one can tell the freshness of a loaf of bread by its softness. On any day you can see housewives pinching loaves of bread on supermarket shelves to see if they're fresh. These shoppers are fooling themselves. Bakers put chemical softeners into the dough that keep the bread soft long after it goes stale.

Another undesirable practice of mass-production bakeries is adding a chemical that keeps within the dough the gases that normally form in the baking process and escape into the air. The result is a loaf of bread that is mostly empty space.

Altogether, there may be 60 additives in the average loaf of bread.

The total result of today's milling and baking processes is the white, soft, nutritionless, tasteless loaf that may justly be described by the epithet at the beginning of this section— tasteless cotton. In his 1957 novel, *Wanda and Hebe*, author Wolfgang Mellors sums it up in a passage concerning a man who "took a puff from his sandwich, then bit on the filter of his cigarette."

Beef—The Weakened Flesh

Not very long ago cattle roamed rangeland, fattening on grass. The fattened cattle were driven to railroad cars and taken to the slaughterhouse. Beef—the flesh of cattle—was as good as nature could make it. Unfortunately, this way of producing meat is all but gone, replaced by artificial methods of reproduction and feeding and doctoring that produce beef faster. And even the packers who buy the quickly fattened cattle admit that they cannot get a good cut of meat from them.

The production of calves is no longer simply a natural process. Frozen bull semen is shipped to cattle raisers who artificially inseminate cows. By manipulating the cows' periods of ovulation with hormones, the time between births is shortened, thus producing more calves.

As soon as a calf is born food additives come into its life. They are in the feed its mother eats. In a previous section we saw that for 27 years the hormone diethylstilbestrol (DES) was put into cattle feed. Some of this chemical enters the cow's milk and then enters the calf's body through nursing.

The cow's feed also contains considerable amounts of antibiotics. These, too, enter the calf's body through its mother's milk. These antibiotics can sensitize the calf so that later, when it begins to eat feed containing antibiotics, it may suffer allergic reactions or die of anaphylactic shock.

At weaning, calves are put into separate feedlots. The young animals walk back and forth along the fence between them and their mothers and bawl continually. This very natural action takes energy. The expenditure of energy causes the calves to lose weight and their anxiety keeps them from the feeding troughs where they should be if they are to gain weight as fast as the cattle raisers want them to. But cattlemen, not to be discouraged, simply give them tranquilizing drugs, which calm them down to the point where they go to the feeding troughs.

Modern cattle feed routinely contains tranquilizers because it has been found that these drugs not only keep the animals quiet in the feedlots, but, for some reason, causes them to eat more. Today, a steer may never be off tranquilizers from the day it is weaned until it goes to slaughter. This has prompted a British physician, Dr. Franklin Bicknell, to question whether or not "feeding young cattle on tranquilizers to increase their rate of growth leaves enough of these mischievous drugs in their meat to affect man." This question has not been fully answered.

The antibiotics in beef animals' feed not only affects the animals themselves, but may affect human beings who eat the beef. In 1967, the FDA said that new information about bacteria that develop resistance to antibiotics given animals and transfer this resistance to humans who consume the animals' meat and milk makes a total ban on some antibiotics advisable. This total ban has not yet been forthcoming, however. In 1969, the British government restricted two antibiotics in cattle feed. A report said, "We do not accept the statement that twenty years of experience goes to show that there are no serious ill-effects from giving antibiotics to animals." Antibiotic-resistant strains of bacteria have developed in the bodies of beef animals. One type of salmonella bacteria has developed such a resistance, and it has been shown that (besides killing many calves) the salmonella infection can be transmitted from calves to man.

The whole idea of modern cattle raising is to put weight on the animals as fast as possible at the least cost possible. Corn-fed steers are as outdated as 78 rpm records. Modern feeds include, along with some proportion of grain, such materials as sawdust and ground newspapers mixed with molasses, cornstarch, corn sugar, corn oil, vitamins, and minerals. In one test, a cow living on a diet of the foregoing ingredients gave birth to a calf that lived to an age of 16 days and suddenly fell dead. An extensive post-mortem failed to turn up the cause of death.

Not long ago, tender beef was produced by hanging a steer carcass in a refrigerator for two to three weeks. As the meat ripened, it also became discolored and shrank a bit. Later, the discoloration had to be trimmed. All this took time, which for the meat packer was money. The process was speeded up by chilling the meat, exposing it to room temperature, then chilling it again. This sequence caused the meat to release the natural enzymes that tenderized it. Best of all, the process took only two days. But this still was not fast enough for the money-hungry packers; warehouse space and handling were also required, and these cost money. To speed up beef tenderizing, enzymes were injected into beef cattle just before slaughter, or right afterward. Then the animal could be cut up and packed without any waiting period for tenderizing. When the injected meat is cooked, the enzymes bromelin from pineapple and papain from papaya act to tenderize it. Neither of these enzymes is known to be harmful to the consumer, but both can disguise tough, stringy meat from elderly bulls or worn-out cows.

The quick fattening of cattle and the quick tenderizing of their meat has been a boon to cattle raisers and meat packers, but not to consumers. The consumer runs the risk of changes in his own metabolism caused by residues of hormones in meat. He also runs the risk of being slowly desensitized to the germ-killing effects of antibiotics. If he suffers a serious wound or a massive bacterial invasion, he will not respond to doses of antibiotics given him by his physician. This is in addition to the allergic sensitization which we have already mentioned. And finally, and far from least, the gains in beef animals' weight for which cattle raisers struggle so hard are made up mainly of watery fat instead of the nutritious protein of healthy beef muscle. Not long ago, a New York congressman told a congressional hearing, "As far as quality is concerned, is it not a fact that there are millions of pounds of meat sold in this country every week which can acquire a taste on your palate only if they are doused with strong sauces? Are we not, in effect, sacrificing a great deal of quality for quantity in our meat supply?"

Assembly-Line Hogs

Hog raising has not escaped the weight-forcing processes. Antibiotics are as common in hog feed as in cattle feed. Copper sulfate has been found to stimulate the growth of hogs. Copper, however, is a heavy metal that can lodge in body tissues and accumulate for years while poisoning the system.

Artificial insemination for sows is not yet quite feasible, but is being worked on. Boar semen cannot be stored for more than a few days. If, during these few days, a sow is not in heat, artificial insemination cannot be carried out. However, a new drug is just about ready for remedying this situation, and if it receives FDA approval, it will be added to the feed of gilts (young cows) to induce a period of heat. Then, fresh boar semen can be used for insemination. If this synchronization can be achieved, it will be, according to *Farm Journal*, "the greatest advance in hog production since the development of antibiotics."

In many states hogs are fed processed garbage. This includes cooked garbage in which heat has destroyed a number of essential amino acids and vitamins. One of the results of this unsavory diet has been stomach ulcers in almost 55 percent of American hogs. Also, garbage is suspected of spreading the deadly diseases cholera, brucellosis, and trichinosis.

The garbage diet plus the poor sanitary conditions in which most hogs are kept adds to the number of diseases that hogs contract. One result is a high mortality of piglets. To overcome this, the piglets may be taken away from the sow shortly after they are born and put into temperature-controlled pens, where they are fed a synthetic diet high in vitamins and minerals. This pulls the weaklings through infancy and frees the sow to be mated again almost immediately. Sows can then be made to bear three litters a year instead of two.

In some modern piggeries, the animals are crowded together so that they can barely move. Moving around uses up energy that burns body fat, and hog raisers want their animals to be as fat as pigs, and even fatter. After a short life in a crowded environment with poor feed and a diet of drugs, a hog is sent to slaughter.

Does all this manipulation stop with the death of a "junkie" pig? No. Prior to or just after slaughter the hog may have tenderizers pumped into its veins.

The result of all this artificial manipulation of the natural growth process is pork that is known to packers as PSE—pale, soft, exudative (watery). Dr. Jonathan Forman, former editor of the *Ohio State Medical Journal*, wrote, "We know . . . that the typical pig ready for market is a sick animal—the victim of obesity—who would die long before his time if we did not rush him to market for the city people to eat."

Mass-Produced Poultry

Poultry suffers the worst of the chemical-filled, computer-directed, short lives of the meat producing animals.

Chicks are hatched by the hundred thousands and kept in trays that afford each barely an inch or two of room in which to move. No sooner is a chick hatched than it is eating antibiotic-laced feed.

Hatcheries sell the chicks to either poultry raisers or egg farms. The poultry raisers are interested in producing broilers for the food market and egg-layers for hatcheries. This is a highly competitive field and every forcing technique available is used. The birds are kept in windowless, temperature-controlled sheds that provide barely enough room for a chicken to stand. Crowding induces nervousness and fighting, and makes the spread of disease almost a certainty. The chicken feed contains tranquilizers, antibiotics, and certain arsenic compounds which speed up maturing, aid the growth of feathers, and give the skin a yellow color. This color is considered more desirable than the pale white skin that results from keeping the chickens in the mass production henhouses. Next time you are in a meat market, compare the yellow skin of some chickens with the pinkish flesh-color of the better grades of broilers—if you can find any.

Government regulations require that the arsenic-containing feed must be discontinued a sufficient time before slaughter so the chickens may eliminate most of the arsenic from their bodies. Although arsenic is considered a carcinogen by the United States Public Health Service, the FDA allows a residue of 0.5 parts per million in chicken flesh. Surveys made by the FDA show that poultry raisers frequently fail to withhold their chickens from market for the required length of time. Dangerous concentrations of arsenic have been found in chickens, especially in the liver, which is the detoxifying organ of animals.

In 1935, a pound of poultry meat was produced over 16 or 17 weeks with five pounds of chicken feed. Today, it takes nine weeks and half as much feed. The feed is very different from that which was used in 1935, and so is the meat. Today's, high-powered, drug-filled chicken feeds produce the same kind of watery-fat meat that modern husbandry methods produce in all other kinds of meat animals.

The All-American Hamburger and Hot Dog

Hot dogs and hamburgers are as American as capitalism, Elvis, and Joe's Bar & Grill. Americans stuff literally billions of them into their hungry faces; in 1971, more than 20 billion hot dogs and hamburgers were consumed in this country. What went into these two meat products was not always something the eaters would lick their lips over.

The simple act of grinding increases the surface of meat, breaks tissues, and releases liquids held in the tissue cells. The ground meat becomes a much more suitable medium for the growth of bacteria than the unground meat was.

Also, grinding makes it easy to conceal exactly what the ground meat actually is or what it's made of. The better hamburger is all beef with no more than 30 percent fat, although less than half that amount of meat is in most kinds. Since there are few state standards for ground meat, almost anything can find its way into hamburger. The poorer grades may contain horse and kangaroo meat; stale meat trimmings; pig hearts, kidneys, and snout muscles; sheep hearts; cattle's lip muscles; and bull testicles.

When ground meat contains a large proportion of fat, it is light pink. Sellers consider this to be an undesirable color, so they may adulterate the meat with cochineal (a red dye from ground insects), coal-tar dyes, or sodium nitrite. This last ingredient is illegal, but it is frequently found in hamburger meat. Sodium nitrite changes in the stomach to nitrous acid, which can cause biological mutations.

Sodium sulfite may be added to hamburger in order to mask the odor of putrefying meat. Besides being toxic, it destroys vitamin B in the foods to which it is added. Still another additive is sodium nicotinate, which gives meat a bright red color. This adulterant, too, is poisonous. Its use is banned in some states, but not in most.

The consumer buying hamburger in a restaurant or "burger joint" is taking his chances on getting good meat. The larger hamburger chains exercise a fair to good amount of control over the quality of their meat, however.

If you are buying hamburger at a butcher shop or meat counter of a supermarket, it is better to stay away from ready ground meat. Next best is to buy a whole cut of beef and have it ground—preferably in your sight, so that you can see the cleanliness of the grinder and watch that no other meat is substituted for that which you bought. Best of all, buy the cut of beef and grind it at home.

The hot dog was introduced into the United States at the Chicago World's Fair of 1893. Its popularity skyrocketed and its reputation for cleanliness plummeted equally fast among those who were in a position to know. Upton Sinclair's description in his novel, *The Jungle*, of the making of frankfurters and other stuffed meats, gave a picture of such filthy conditions that it led to the passage of the Federal Meat Inspection Act of

1906. Today, frankfurters* sold in interstate commerce must be federally inspected. Those not sold across state lines are regulated by state law which may be enforced laxly. About one-third of all frankfurters are not federally inspected.

The USDA limits to 10 per cent any water added to hot dog meat. In frankfurters made at processing plants not inspected by the government, a water content of more than 60 per cent has been found. There is a federal limit of 30 per cent for fat, but some frankfurters may be as much as one-half fat. Many hot dogs contain extenders—materials that add bulk. Among these are starch, cereals, and nonfat dry milk. These are not harmful, but they cheat consumers who believe they are buying a meat product. It is a misrepresentation in law for hot dogs labeled "all meat" or "all beef" to contain extenders. "All meat" frankfurters are not necessarily as good a buy as they may seem. The meat may include a high proportion of cattle, hog, and chicken parts that most people would rather not eat. The best buy is federally inspected all-beef hot dogs.

The poorer of the foregoing ingredients may not be nutritional or very pleasant-tasting (although bad taste is usually well masked with spices), but they are harmless. However, a large proportion of hot dogs are colored with dyes that are known to be harmful (and illegal) or whose harmlessness has not been definitely established. It is the frankfurter casing that is dyed, not the meat, but there are far too many poor quality casings which "bleed" their color into the meat. Other definitely or possibly harmful ingredients in hot dogs are antioxidants, tenderizers, and rancidity retarders.

Fresh Fish?

Fish once were in the regular diet of only those people living

---

* In Germany and Austria each city has its own meat specialty. Though the hot dog bears no resemblance to these excellent meats, it still carries several of their names— Hamburger, Frankfurter, Wiener (Vienna).

near oceans or other large bodies of water. With the invention of ice-making machinery and the refrigerated railway car, fish could be transported to consumers living far inland. Unfortunately, this transportation was not always successful. When trains were delayed, ice melted; when refrigeration machinery broke down, the insides of railway cars warmed up. In either case, the warmed fish spoiled. Then, after World War II, quick freezing came into wide use, and the transporting of unspoiled fish to any part of the country seemed to be solved. But it was soon found that quick freezing brought its own problems.

Freezing, unlike canning, does not stop the action of natural enzymes in fish. The longer the fish remains frozen, the greater are the results of the enzymes' actions. When old frozen fish is thawed, it exudes a thick, watery liquid; the flesh is dry and tough, and may be yellowish or brownish; it has a rancid smell and usually is tasteless, or it may have an unpleasant taste. In one survey of supermarkets, United States Department of the Interior inspectors found frozen fish as much as *four years* old.

It is not unusual for frozen fish to be allowed accidently to thaw when in storage or transit. When this happens the fish is refrozen slowly in distributors' or dealers' refrigerators. Slow freezing breaks the cell walls of the flesh, and when the fish is thawed, it is in much the same condition as frozen fish spoiled by enzyme action.

The public soon became aware of the shortcomings of frozen fish and began to stay away from it. The frozen fish industry had the answer to this problem—additives. Since the action that spoils fish includes bacterial enzymes, it is simple to dip the fish in antibiotic solutions before freezing. Then, when the dealer gets the frozen fish, he thaws it and puts it into his display counter as "fresh fish." The antibiotic dip is perfectly legal; it has been permitted by the FDA since 1959, even though dipped fish may contain up to five parts per million of antibiotic residue. Haddock treated with antibiotics and kept on ice in a dealer's showcase will remain "fresh" for 25 days; red snappers, 30 days, and scallops, 22 days.

Advocates of antibiotic dipping claim that cooking destroys all the antibiotics except a small amount which is "of no medical significance." However, this residue added to antibiotic residues in other foods can total an amount of definite medical significance.

The fishing industry is allowed to preserve fish in transit by packing it in ice that contains sodium nitrite, sodium benzoate, ozone, hydrogen peroxide, or chlorine as preservatives. Sodium nitrite, as we have seen, is a dangerous additive, and the others are highly undesirable.

It might be well to note here that a fish which is truly fresh is hard to get. Today, a fish may be not long out of water but it is rarely fresh in the sense of being untainted and healthful. The reason is simple: there are very few unpolluted bodies of water in which the fish could have lived. Even the oceans, far from shore, are fouled with pesticides. Natural waters near ocean shores and those of rivers and lakes are polluted with industrial wastes and sewerage, as well as pesticides. Fish are sensitive to these pollutants and are killed by the millions. More important to the consumer, pesticides and other pollutants are stored in the fatty tissues of fish. It is the rule, rather than the exception, to find fish with more DDT in their flesh than is considered safe for human consumption. Also, in 1971, several investigators both in and out of government reported that industrial wastes had for years been contaminating fish, as well as shellfish, crabs, lobsters, and shrimp with mercury. This metal is very poisonous, and causes brain damage.

Milk—Babies Beware!

The word "milk" brings to mind contented cows in lush green buttercup-speckled fields, happy babies, and healthy children. That's what the dairy industry's endless and massive promotion wants you to think. Milk, we are told, is the "nearly perfect food." "Milk is food for every member of your family." You are told to "drink three glasses of milk a day" all your life because "you never outgrow your need for milk."

Milk once was a nutritious food, but it is no longer what it was, nor are the cows that produce it. Gone is the contented cow. Elsie has been replaced by a nervous milk-producing junkie that is routinely fed tranquilizers. She may never walk in a buttercup-speckled field (sigh!)—but let's not cry over spilled milk. Instead, she spends her whole life in a huge barn, walking on exercising treadmills and eating antibiotic-laced feeds in place of grass. She has been bred to have an udder so utterly large that she does not look much like the storybook cow. However, she produces thousands of gallons more milk a year.

Penicillin has become a part of a modern dairy cow's diet. It is commonly used to combat mastitis, an inflammation of the udder that is a widespread ailment of cows. Penicillin is also fed to cows to keep the bacterial count in milk low. The antibiotic does its job, but a considerable residue of it remains in the milk. This can be a serious matter to milk drinkers who are allergic to penicillin. Doctors know that they must not prescribe penicillin indiscriminately, yet it is distributed in that manner to milk drinkers.

Hormones are administered to cows to increase their production of milk. The hormones, of course, get into the milk and may upset the hormone balance of milk drinkers. One hormone, estrin, produced female sex characteristics in men who drank milk from a dairy where the hormone was being used.

Milk-inspection authorities continually warn dairies about detergents in milk. The detergents get into milk when washed milk cans are incompletely rinsed. A large amount of detergent in his milk could make a consumer ill, but even relatively small amounts can kill beneficial bacteria that are especially valuable when the milk is used to make cheese or cultured milk.

As mentioned previously, insufficiently refined paraffin used to coat cardboard milk containers may contain a known cancer-producing substance, 1,2,5,6 dibenzanthracene. When this fact was announced, some dairies switched to polyethylene milk containers, but most milk still comes in wax-coated cartons. The danger here is not from properly refined wax coating, but as long as a milk container may be coated with insufficiently refined wax, the consumer is forced to play Russian roulette with a known carcinogen.

Milk, like almost all other kinds of food today, contains pesticide residues. Almost all milk contains some of the radioactive isotope strontium-90, which can produce genetic damage. It gets into milk via fallout from the testing of nuclear weapons. The fallout is carried to earth in raindrops and enters plants through their roots. Plants eaten as fodder by cows carry strontium-90 into cows' digestive systems, from where it enters the milk. With above-ground nuclear testing almost eliminated, the menace of strontium-90 lessens with time but will remain serious for many years. The only mitigating factor in the tragic situation of a radioactive element in milk is that calcium, also in milk, cuts down the incorporation of strontium-90 into bones.

With dairymen's efforts aimed at higher quantities (if not higher quality) of milk, overproduction was inevitable. They attacked the problem in several ways. One was to popularize the drinking of skim milk as a way of cutting down on the number of calories in one's diet. They also pushed skim milk as an ingredient in non-fat ice cream, cheese, pie fillings, and other products aimed at the overweight consumer.

To obtain skim milk, whole milk is run through a separator which removes the butterfat. The fraction that is left, the skim milk, is minus vitamins A, D, E, and K, which remain in the fat. The nutritional value of skim milk is considerably less than whole milk.

Another way of using up overproduced milk is to make nonfat dry milk. There are two processes by which this milk product is made. In spray drying, the butterfat is first removed and then the remaining milk is pasteurized. Then it is partly evaporated. Finally, it is blown through nozzles into vacuum chambers. The remaining nonfat milk powder has most of the nutritional elements of milk minus fat and a few vitamins.

The second method of making nonfat dry milk is to let the fat-free milk flow over heated metal drums. This process quickly evaporates the water, leaving flakes of dried milk which are then powdered. The high heat necessary to evaporate the water rapidly destroys important proteins and vitamins, leaving a nutritionally poor product. Laboratory animals fed nonfat dry milk made by the drum-drying process died of protein deficiency diseases. It is not necessary by law for the manufacturer to label his product with the kind of drying process he uses, so consumers should press the FDA for a regulation making such labeling mandatory.

Evaporated, or condensed, milk has had some of its water removed by a special process that increases the storage life of the remaining milk. Unfortunately, the water is removed from protein molecules, thus debasing the nutritive value of the milk. Also, vitamin B_6 is destroyed.

Dr. Francis M. Pottinger, Jr., reported in the *Journal of Orthodontics and Oral Surgery* on an experiment in feeding cats raw milk and milk treated in various ways. The cats that fed on raw milk flourished and died of old age; those fed evaporated milk developed protein deficiency diseases and died young. Another study reported that infants fed evaporated milk suffered convulsions until vitamin B_6 was added to the milk.

Although condensed milk has a long shelf life, especially when refrigerated, it does deteriorate. To slow this process, a number of additives are permitted in the milk, among them calcium chloride, disodium phosphate, sodium citrate, vitamin D, and carrageenan. To enhance the flavor of the milk, refined sugar and/or refined corn syrup is added.

Modern butter suffers from the deficiencies of the milk that goes into making it, and has some undesirable characteristics of its own added. Butter may be bleached with hydrogen peroxide, have NDGA added as an antioxidant, have acidity neutralized by any one of several alkaline chemicals, and contain salt as a preservative. When butter was made from fresh, unadulterated milk, it changed color with the seasons. In the cold months, butter was light yellow, almost white; in the warmer part of the year, it was a deeper yellow. The reason for the change was that in the warmer months, cows ate yellow flowers, such as buttercups, and the coloring matter (carotene) of the flowers imparted color to the butter. Now, synthetic carotene (a harmless dye) and a number of coal-tar dyes keep butter yellow all year around. Some of these yellow dyes were definitely shown to be cancer-producing before they were banned; some now being used are of very questionable safety.

Cheeses, too, carry on the deficiencies of the milk that goes into them. The Microbiological Section of the Canadian Food and Drug Directorate warned: "Where penicillin or other antibiotics are used with dairy cattle, the survival of resistant [bacterial] organisms may lead to widespread distribution of resistant strains into the homes of the general populace, since *staphylococci* and *streptococci*, often in large numbers, are of common occurrence in cheese." What do the cheese makers do about these staph and strep germs? Add more and different antibiotics, of course, to suppress the germs in your cheese.

Cottage cheese, an unaged cheese made by coagulating whey, is a happy hunting ground for bacteria, molds, and yeasts. Luckily, most of these are harmless, but they make the cheese taste bad. So, into cottage cheese go stabilizers for uniform thickness and color, smooth texture, and desirable flavor. Mold inhibitors give longer shelf life. Despite these additives, inspection continually finds containers of cottage cheese with undesirably high bacterial and mold counts.

Ice cream can be a healthful food. It can be made of milk,

sugar, gelatin, eggs, fruits, nuts, and natural colors. Instead, almost all modern ice cream is a dumping ground for almost every kind of stabilizer, antioxidant, preservative, filler, moisture control, and artificial color and flavor known to food processing. According to FDA regulations, the only information that need appear on a package of ice cream is the name of the product (ice cream), the flavor, and whether the flavor is artificial. In view of the number of additives in ice cream, this lax regulation is a complete failure on the part of the FDA to perform its function of protecting the consumer.

Sugar—a Not-So-Sweet Story

Sugar can be made by crushing sugar cane, extracting the sap, and slowly evaporating this liquid. Sugar can also be made in much the same manner from the juice of the sugar beet. The evaporated sap of maple trees in late winter is another source of sugar. These three kinds of sugar are natural and have nutritive values, including calcium, iron, phosphorus, sodium, potassium, and vitamins A, B_1, B_2, B_3, D, E, and pantothenic acid; also the trace elements, copper, zinc, manganese, and iron in an easily assimilable form. White, refined, granulated sugar lacks all these items except very small amounts of sodium and potassium, the least valuable from the standpoint of nutrition.

Many people believe that brown sugar is more healthful than white sugar. Actually, brown sugar may be less healthful. The brown color is not natural; it comes from a residue of the bone charcoal with which the sugar was boiled. This process gets rid of the much darker color of molasses, most of which was previously removed from the raw sugar. Dr. Heuper, the cancer expert, says, "In themselves, sugars may not be carcinogenic—but carcinogenic impurities may be introduced into sugars when concentrated sugar solutions are filtered for decolorizing purposes through improperly prepared charcoal containing polycyclic hydrocarbons. . . . Traces [of these hydrocarbons] may remain in apparently chemically pure sugars."

The United States has a higher per capita consumption of sugar than any other country. It is estimated conservatively that each person uses a quarter of a pound of sugar *each day*. "Sugar must be one of our most needed foods—that's why we like it so much," the Sugar Institute advertises. Nutritionists think otherwise. Dr. Michael H. Walsh, instructor in clinical nutrition at the University of California, writes, "When it comes to human diets, there is no object in furnishing sugar unless appropriate amounts of proteins, fats, minerals, and vitamins are also furnished. Refined sugar, because of its highly concentrated form, and being completely devoid of essential proteins, vitamins, and minerals, is now regarded nutritionally as a diluting agent of the modern diet. It is a displacer of other factors far more essential than sugar. Thus, the more sugar consumed, the less opportunity for getting essential nutrients into the diet. If sugar is furnished as a replacement of proteins, fats, minerals, and vitamins, then serious physiological consequences follow. This is the essence and the crux of the physiological problem we have to deal with, not only in dentistry, but also in medicine."

"Eat sugar for 'quick energy' " is another urging of the sugar interests. Is this true? Barely, and at a price, says Dr. John Yudkin, Emeritus Professor of Nutrition at London University. "Normally you have quite a sizable reserve of . . . fuel in your tissues, stored from the food you have eaten on previous occasions. If you were starving so that you had little or none of these reserves, and if in addition it were imperative that you have some fuel in your tissues within minutes, in addition to the glucose in your blood, then it might be a good idea to eat sugar rather than any other food, because sugar quickly gets digested and absorbed and taken to the tissues. A piece of bread and butter would take a few minutes longer." Dr. Yudkin continues, "All other foods contain energy as well as at least *some* nutrients in the way of protein or minerals or vitamins or a mixture of these. Sugar contains energy, and that is all." Other nutritionists have pointed out that the sudden ingestion of sugar can raise the blood-sugar level temporarily, and then let it fall dangerously below the normal level.

Maple syrup has long been considered to be a healthfully pure product, but man in his wisdom has managed to change this, too. Certain bacteria that are normally found in a maple tree slow down the flow of sap. It has been found that a pellet of paraformaldehyde, placed at the tap hole, will kill the bacteria. These pellets, which are long-lasting, also keep the tap holes open longer, thus increasing the sap flow and making more profit for the maple grove owner.

The FDA has sanctioned the use of the paraformaldehyde pellet, whereas the Canadian Food and Drug Directorate has refused to allow the use of the pellet, although there is a large maple sugar industry in Canada. Many maple grove owners in the United States, however, refuse to use the pellet because they feel that maple sugar and maple syrup have a reputation for purity that should be preserved.

The pellet allows the tree to be tapped earlier than normal. In January, the tree's internal chemistry is producing growth substances which mix with the sap, giving it a "buddy" taste. To overcome this, a culture of bacteria *(Pseudomonas geniculata)* is added to the "buddy"-tasting maple syrup and is allowed to ferment. This disguises the unwanted taste, and the product can be sold as "pure maple syrup."

Honey is the ideal substitute for the refined packaged sugars. It contains three sugars: sucrose (cane sugar), dextrose (grape sugar), and levulose (fruit sugar). The first of these is present in a small amount; the other two are very easily assimilated and stored in the body. Honey also contains proteins, vitamins, and minerals.

Pure honey, right out of the honeycomb, is slightly cloudy. Most consumers are not aware of this fact, taking the cloudiness to be an impurity. Because of this, honey may be heated and filtered. The heating destroys some of the vitamins, but heated and clarified honey is still an excellent source of sugar.

Honey production has become big business, and with this development have come the abuses that usually accompany the drive for large profits. To extract honey from the comb, some bees must be gotten out of the way. This formerly was a slow process. Now, irritating chemicals are used to do the job quickly. Among them are phenol (carbolic acid), benzaldehyde, propionic anhydride, and nitrous oxide. To stave off bee diseases, antibiotics and sulfa drugs are used. Empty hives may be fumigated with methyl bromide or paradichlorobenzene (moth-ball material). Any of these substances may find its way into honey and contaminate it.

Baby Foods—Off to a Wrong Start in Life

Baby foods are subject to all the contamination, false promotion, and callous disregard for the ultimate consumer (in this case, the baby) that adult foods are.

A baby's first food is, of course, milk. In the United States, where only a minority of infants are breast fed, the majority are bottle fed with so-called infant formulas. Most formulas are made up of cow's milk with one or more kinds of sugar added.

Cow's milk has approximately three times as much protein and half as much carbohydrate (in the form of lactose, or milk sugar) as human milk. To lower the protein content, cow's milk is simply diluted with water. The necessary additional lactose is then added—or at least it should be added. Instead, many formula manufacturers add maltose (malt sugar), dextrose (grape sugar), or ordinary table sugar. An infant's digestive system cannot assimilate these sugars as easily as lactose.

In 1966, the *Wall Street Journal* reported that there were about 156 infant formulas on the market; today, there are more. In some, Coca-Cola syrup and strawberry Jell-o are added to combat diarrhea. Others have goat's milk for babies allergic to cow's milk. There are many additives put into infant formulas allegedly for nutritional purposes or to combat digestive difficulties. Most of these are useless and some are directly harmful. Even the useless ones do harm because they deny nourishment to the infant. It is especially important that infant formulas be pure and without any additives that are even mildly toxic, because an infant's bodily system does not have the fully functioning detoxifying mechanisms found in adults.

The infant formula manufacturers have very stiff competition from the manufacturers of solid baby foods. The latter urge mothers to put their babies on solid food as soon as possible. According to leading baby specialists, the solid food manufacturers are becoming successful, which is alarming. Feeding a baby solid food too soon can deny it needed nourishment. Before the age of six months, infants' saliva does not contain ptyalin, the enzyme that digests starch. Furthermore, the pancreatic gland, which completes the digestion of starch, does not develop until a baby's molar teeth erupt. Until then, the undigested starch may ferment, causing rashes, indigestion, and even respiratory ailments. Nonetheless, cereals, pablum, and processed rice and mashed potatoes are among infant foods pushed by their makers. And many baby foods contain starch in the form of white flour.

A great variety of chicken, meat, vegetable, fruit, and pudding preparations are sold as baby foods. Manufacturers learned that many mothers choose baby foods on the basis of what they themselves like. So, spices, flavors, and salt that are useless or harmful to the baby are added to the baby foods. Salt is especially dangerous. Well documented studies have shown that babies fed more salt than naturally appears in food have a very high expectation of developing hypertension later in life. A survey revealed that the amount of salt in processed baby foods is about twice as high as in nonprocessed foods. The investigators noted that the addition of salt in amounts excessive in relation to a baby's needs was done to make the baby foods more palatable to the mothers.

In 1962, the UN's Food and Health Organization of the World Health Organization issued a report that summed up the baby food problem as follows:

"Foods that are specifically prepared for babies require separate considerations from all other foods as regards the use of food additives and toxicological risks. The reason for this is that the detoxicating mechanisms that are effective in the more mature individual may be ineffective in the baby. The committee strongly urges that baby foods should be prepared without food additives, if possible. If the use of a food additive is necessary in a baby food, great caution should be exercised both in the choice of the additive and the level of use."

Very few, if any, manufacturers of baby foods in the United States adhere very strictly to the FAO/WHO warning.

The Almost Impossible Task

As noted before, it is almost impossible to buy foods that are not contaminated or nutritionally debased by food additives. We have seen how this applies to flour, bread, beef, pork, poultry, processed meats, milk and milk products, sugar, and baby foods. These are the basic foods, but almost all the other foods on grocers' shelves have been processed in ways that diminish their natural nourishment or toxify them. The crops grown by organic farmers or manufactured by health food companies cannot begin to fulfill the volume of demand of the American consumer. There is no place to turn for healthful foods. We are forced to pollute our bodies.

Surrogate Nutrition— Synthetics and Substitutes

Food technologists have not stopped at adulterating foods with additives. They have gone on to the ultimate in debasing food: wholly synthetic foodstuffs fabricated without any help from nature.

In 1965, the magazine *Soviet Life* reported a triumph of Russian chemists in bringing the good life to the consumer: synthetic caviar. This product, the magazine says, is "absolutely indistinguishable from the natural variety . . . it takes a microscope to see the difference." The writer of this article did not say what the artificial sturgeon eggs were made of, and perhaps it was a good thing he did not—the ersatz caviar fancier might not enjoy his delicacy if he knew what went into it. One thing is highly probable—the synthetic caviar lacked the natural vitamins A and D found in fish eggs.

Surprisingly, synthetic caviar has yet to make a place for itself on the shelves of American supermarkets, but some of our food chemists have promised us a host of other ersatz goodies. We will have peas made of starch and a binder, colored and flavored—no doubt with synthetic colors and flavors. So-called spun vegetable proteins, plus fats, flavors, and colors all held together with binders, will provide simulated meats, poultry, and fish.

Synthetic Milk

One synthetic foodstuff that has become very widely used is synthetic milk or synthetic cream, whichever you prefer to call it. It is also called "non-dairy creamer." Whatever its name, it has no connection with cows. It is made of corn syrup, water, a hydrogenated vegetable oil, sodium caseinate (from soybeans or milk solids), potassium phosphate, emulsifier, stabilizer, salt, synthetic vitamins and minerals, and artificial flavors and colors.

The manufacturers of synthetic milk say that their product has advantages over cow's milk. Because it is less vulnerable to the action of bacteria, it has a longer shelf life. Its flavor is more stable. It meets the requirements of Jewish dietary laws for being a non-milk food. Most important, synthetic milk is cheaper to produce than cow's milk. A quart of imitation milk costs about two-thirds as much to produce as a quart of cow's milk. Non-dairy creamer and synthetic whipping cream cost about half as much as natural cream and whipping cream.

The producers of synthetic milk loudly point out that their product lacks the saturated butterfat of milk, which like all saturated fats is suspected of being a cause of hypertension and heart trouble. However, the butterfat is replaced by hydrogenated fats, such as coconut oil. According to Drs. E. R. Monsen and L. Adriaenssens, writing in the *American Journal of Clinical Nutrition*, the hydrogenated fats contain a higher percentage of saturated fatty acids than are found in butterfat. Other scientists writing in the same publication said that synthetic milks "are in no sense a nutritional replacement for milk in proteins, minerals, and vitamins." They found the protein content of several brands of synthetic milk to vary from below to above that of cow's milk. The brands with higher protein content were not a boon to the consumer because the proteins were of the type the body has difficulty in using. Still other investigators said that "the imitation milks . . . as formulated today are unsuitable for infants and children . . . from the standpoint of low content of protein, essential amino acids, and minerals." And these milk products were agreed to be "potentially harmful for other vulnerable age groups such as pregnant and lactating women, and persons on marginal diets such as those in low income groups and the aged."

Margarine—Synthetic Butter

Margarine is usually composed of vegetable oils which are hardened to the consistency of butter by the process of hydrogenation. The oils most commonly used are corn, cottonseed, and soybean; however, if at any time animal fats are cheaper, some of these will be mixed with the vegetable oils. In the hydrogenation process, the oils are raised to a high temperature in the presence of a catalyst such as nickel or platinum, then hydrogen gas is bubbled through the oils. This process opens up most of the double or triple chemical bonds between the carbon atoms of the fatty acids that make up the oils. Hydrogen atoms attach themselves to these open bonds in an action known as saturation, a process that is carried out only to the point at which the oils take on the consistency of butter. In the case of margarine, saturation is not complete. This means that some of the chemical bonds remain unsaturated, and the margarine fat is said to be *polyunsaturated.*

In the early 1960's, experimental evidence seemed to point to the fact that unsaturated fats are healthier for the consumer than those that are saturated. There is still much disagreement among scientists about this conclusion. However, producers of margarine saw a way to exploit the possibility that unsaturated fats are nutritionally better. It was an especially good time to do this because the average person had become very conscious of the epidemic proportions of high blood pressure and heart disease, both of which were linked to fatty deposits in the arteries. The margarine manufacturers advertised that since their product was made of vegetable oils, it was an unsaturated fat and therefore would prevent circulatory system diseases. They conveniently left out mention of the hydrogenation process. What the hardening process does to the fatty acids in margarine is explained by Dr. Franklin Bicknell in *Chemicals in Food and in Farm Produce: Their Harmful Effects*:

"The abnormal fatty acids produced by 'hardening' [hydrogenation] are the real worry. The atoms of the molecule of an essential fatty acid [EFA] are arranged in space in a particular manner . . . but hardening may produce a different spatial arrangement, so that a completely abnormal . . . unsaturated fatty acid is produced. An analogy is ordinary handwriting and mirror handwriting: both are identical but spatially different, so that at best reading the latter is difficult and at worst serious mistakes are made. The same mistakes are made by the body when presented . . . [with hydrogenated] EFAs. Not only does it fail to benefit by them, but it is deluded by their similarity to normal EFA and so attempts to use them. It starts incorporating them in biochemical reactions and then finds they are the wrong shape; but the reaction has gone too far to jettison them and begin again with normal EFA, so they are not only useless but actually prevent the use of normal EFA. They are in fact *anti*-EFA. They accentuate in man and animals a deficiency of EFA. An analogy is jamming the wrong key in a lock; not only is the lock not turned but the right key also is rendered valueless." Dr. Ancel Keys warns that the distorted shapes of polyunsaturated fat molecules "are biologically less desirable."

The hydrogenation process gives margarine makers an incidental benefit. Saturated fats cannot become rancid. In order that a food turn rancid, it must be able to combine with oxygen of the air. Since the bonds of saturated fatty acids have all been taken up by hydrogen atoms, there are no places for oxygen atoms to join the hardened fats. Since the fatty acids of margarine are not completely saturated, they can take on some oxygen molecules. As a result margarine takes a long time to become rancid. It has a long storage and shelf-life. This is good for the producer, bad for the consumer. As Dr. Bicknell says, "Food that cannot go bad is bad food."

The metal catalyst used in the hydrogenation process can do considerable harm to the body if not entirely removed from the fat. First, nickel is suspected of being a carcinogen. Second, the nickel can replace certain other metals normally in the body's enzyme system. One investigator has found evidence that the replacement by nickel of at least one metal can cause a pyrodoxine (vitamin B_6) deficiency, and this can lead to atherosclerosis, or hardening of the arteries.

Besides polyunsaturated fats, margarine may contain skim milk or nonfat dry milk solids, water, and ground soybeans. To make margarine as much like "the high priced spread" as possible, a number of additives are incorporated. The hydrogenated fat is white, so it is colored with a yellow dye. In an attempt to render any nickel residue harmless, a metal scavenger, stearyl citrate, is added. Since the fat is not entirely saturated and some rancidity can develop, an antioxidant, butylated hydroxy anisole, may be added. A butterlike flavor and odor are obtained with diacetyl, and are protected with isopropyl citrate. Lethicin gives margarine the frying properties of butter. Putting all these things together is made easier with mono- and/or diglycerides. Finally, the margarine is "enriched" with synthetic vitamins and preserved with citric acid, sodium benzoate, or benzoic acid—the latter two definitely known to be harmful.

A final warning on the ersatz butter is sounded by Dr. Bicknell. "It is difficult to resist the conclusion," he says, "that our increasing arterial degeneration is not the inevitable concomitant of old age, which it may antecede by many years or never join at all, but a preventable pandemic disease of modern foods and especially of modern bread, milk, and margarine."

Lethal Sugar Substitutes

In 1856, an English chemist, William Henry Perkin, made mauve dye from coal tar. This was the first of literally thousands of dyes, paints, lacquers, perfumes, preservatives, solvents, flavorings, and other useful things that have come from coal tar. All these things were produced much more cheaply than their natural predecessors. Food producers welcomed the dyes and flavors, and these became common food additives. Many have been shown to be poisonous and have been banned, but scores are still being used, although their safety is very doubtful.

Another coal-tar product that was welcomed by food processors was saccharin, a sweetener, synthesized in 1879. Saccharin is intensely sweet; a pill the size of a large pinhead is enough to sweeten a cup of coffee. Saccharin is cheap and much less bulky to handle than sugar. All these characteristics rendered it appealing to the food industry, which used it in bakery products, soft drinks, and candies. Eleven years after saccharin was discovered, the French Commission of the Health Association banned its manufacture or import. And in 1898, the German government forbade its use in food and drink. A number of other governments followed suit, but almost a century after its discovery, saccharin was still being used in the United States.

Literally hundreds of scientific papers were written demonstrating the damage to the blood done by saccharin. In 1951, FDA researchers linked the sweetener to cancer. In 1969, another study, this one by Dr. George T. Bryan, an expert on cancerous tumors, reported that saccharin had produced cancer of the bladder in half of each of two groups of mice. Dr. Bryan admitted that he had not established a direct link between saccharin and cancer in man, but he was "very suspicious." He said, "It may take many years before it is known exactly how dangerous the substance is, and until then its use should be restricted to those who need it for medical reasons."

In 1970, after the FDA had put severe limitations on another type of sweetener, the cyclamates, the National Academy of Sciences reviewed saccharin for the FDA. The NAS group concluded that saccharin did "not pose a hazard." But some FDA officials felt that there still were safety questions that needed resolution. By the autumn of 1970, the FDA finally got around to putting restrictions on the use of saccharin.

Although very sweet and convenient, saccharin has some disadvantages. It loses sweetness in canning, cooking, and baking, and it leaves a bitter aftertaste. In 1950, chemists came up with another type of sweetener which overcame the disadvantages of saccharin—cyclamates. Cyclamates maintained their sweetness in food processing and had no aftertaste. They were 30 times as sweet as sugar and cost only one-tenth as much. They seemed to be an answer to food processors' prayers.

Cyclamates appeared on the market at just about the time that Americans became extremely weight conscious, so cyclamate manufacturers aimed their biggest advertising guns at those who wanted to reduce their weight. Cyclamates were quickly crammed into jellies, jams, preserved fruits, ice cream and ice cream cones, sodas, juices, candies, cookies, breakfast cereals, "900 calorie" meals, colas and other "diet" drinks, puddings, syrups, vegetable soups, salad dressings, and bread.

Faced with this flood of uses, the FDA requested the Food Protection Committee, Food and Nutrition Board (National Academy of Sciences–National Research Council) to review the safety of artificial sweeteners. The Committee said, in 1955, that the toxicity of the sweeteners should be known, and that "there has not been extensive controlled studies of the use by people in various physiological states." Then, after these admissions of lack of definite knowledge, the Committee concluded cautiously, "There is no evidence that the use of non-nutritive sweeteners, saccharine and cyclamate, for special dietary purposes is hazardous." The conclusion did not seem to address itself to the question, since cyclamates were being used widely and indiscriminately, not only for "special dietary purposes."

Consumer Reports told how cyclamate manufacturers turned the report around in weasel-worded advertisements. "Non-nutritive" became "no calories." "Should be used only by" was changed to "recommended for," and "for those who must restrict" was twisted to "by persons who desire."

In 1962, the Food Protection Committee was asked by the FDA to make another review of artificial sweeteners. Again, the substitutes were approved, but the Committee cautioned that "the question of the safety of cyclamate for all classes of people is not settled. . . ." And the Committee again said that there was not enough known about the "continued ingestion" of cyclamates in large amounts. Finally, "the priority of public welfare over all other considerations precludes, therefore, the uncontrolled distribution of foodstuffs containing cyclamates." This conclusion would seem to call for restriction, if not total ban, of the general use of cyclamates, but the FDA did not see it that way. Instead, the use of the synthetic sweetener was extended to new groups of foods. In 1967, an estimate placed three-quarters of the population as users of non-nutritive sweeteners.

In the next few years, medical evidence of harm done by cyclamates continued to grow. Damage to fetuses; diarrhea; inhibited growth; damage to kidneys, liver, the intestinal tract, thyroid and adrenal glands; change in blood-coagulation factors that interfered with blood-coagulant drugs; and blocking of the action of antibiotics were some of the adverse actions of cyclamates.

Again, in 1967 this time, the FDA asked the Food Protection Committee to review synthetic sweeteners. The Committee reported that "totally unrestricted use of cyclamates is not warranted at this time." In February 1969, the FDA said it planned to remove cyclamates from the Generally Recognized As Safe (GRAS) list. Late in 1969, evidence that heavy and continued doses of cyclamates caused bladder cancers in rats caused the Secretary of Health, Education, and Welfare to ban the use of cyclamates for general use and to take them off the GRAS list.

The Secretary's action set off a struggle between the manufacturers and those in government who wished to protect the public welfare. The cyclamate manufacturers howled so loudly that the Secretary reclassified cyclamates as drugs instead of food additives. They could then be sold as over-the-counter nonprescription drugs. This did not keep cyclamates out of food. The FDA allowed the sale of cyclamates in liquid or tablet form and also in cyclamate-containing foods if the companies filed abbreviated new applications, without the usual safety and efficiency warranties. The companies simply had to agree to food labels that showed the cyclamate content of an average serving.

The FDA's Medical Advisory Group on Cyclamates had gathered data which demonstrated that foods containing cyclamates were of no use in reducing diets. In fact, laboratory animals gained weight when fed cyclamates in amounts equivalent to those consumed by human beings. With this evidence in hand, the FDA imposed a total ban on cyclamates, but let the existing stocks be sold. Thus, 19 years after the introduction of cyclamates, and about 14 years after evidence of their harmfulness was revealed, this dangerous synthetic food additive was banned.

The United States Department of Agriculture has developed a natural sweetener that could be a substitute for saccharin and cyclamates. It is hesperidin, a natural ingredient in citrus fruits. Since a government department developed the new sweetener, it cannot be patented by any manufacturer. For this reason, no company, so far, is interested in making it.

The banning of saccharin and cyclamates from general use

in food processing are two victories for those who fight against the pollution of the human body by a flood of chemicals, some of which are in the form of wholly artificial foods.

Pollution by Cosmetics
and Drugs

Foods are not the only source of body pollution. Cosmetics and drugs, too, contain numbers of harmful substances. There are numerous kinds of skin creams, body lotions, hair dyes and conditioners, face powders, rouges, lipsticks, and other cosmetics that contain chemical ingredients which injure the skin and abuse the hair. Among drugs, many patent medicines and some prescription drugs are actually poisonously harmful.

Every society has its norms of personal appearance which are called physical beauty. In one society, beauty may consist of large bamboo discs inserted into the upper and lower lips; in another, a well greased body and hair plastered with cow dung makes one beautiful; in modern western culture, beauty is smooth, clear skin, rosy cheeks, lips colored red, pink, orange, silver, or whatever other color is the fashion, and hair that is thick, lustrous, soft-looking, and any color but gray. Since not everyone's skin, cheeks, lips, and hair meet the standards of current beauty norms, changing these physical attributes to meet the norms is the accepted practice. The substances used to achieve the changes are cosmetics.

The Skin Game

The natural, untouched skin of most persons is adequate to perform its functions of surrounding the body with a protective covering and to regulate body temperature. And most skins are pleasant looking. But the hammering of massive advertising has made the average person feel that she or he must look like the photographers' models who appear on television. Also, advertising's accent on youth has made the normal changes in aging skin seem entirely undesirable and unnecessary.

For those with dry or oily skins there are a great number of creams and lotions. The creams for dry skins contain as their basic ingredients glycerine, lanolin, or petrolatum, or a combination of these. Glycerine absorbs moisture from the air, thus keeping dry skins moist. Lanolin and petrolatum cover the dry skin with a thin layer of grease, thereby replacing the skin oils that are lacking in dry skin. Lotions for oily skins contain detergents which temporarily wash away the excess skin oils. Most skin creams and lotions also contain many substances (excluding perfumes) which are useless, but which have sales appeal. The wise consumer who wishes to treat dry skin can save much money by simply buying glycerine or petrolatum in a drugstore and using them *sparingly*. Oily skins washed with mild soap and then *rinsed thoroughly*, will be temporarily cleansed of oil as thoroughly as by the most expensive cosmetic preparation.

Dryness or oiliness of the skin usually is the result of improper diet or imbalance of the body's endocrine system. Curing these skin conditions are medical, not cosmetic, matters. One must learn the proper diet or get the advice of a competent endocrinologist.

If aging causes changes in the skin—dryness, wrinkles, diminished elasticity, and freckling—why not try to reverse the aging process? Diminished production of sex hormones is one of the normal processes of aging, so, says Dr. Cosmetic Advertising, all we have to do is to put some of these hormones on the skin and it will turn back to its youthful condition. Unfortunately, this does not work.

The main hormones included in skin creams are estrogens, an important group of female sex hormones. Very little of the hormones are absorbed by the skin. Dr. Howard Behrman, writing in the *Journal of the American Medical Association*, said that hormone creams do nothing at all for the skin. He pointed out that aging women who have had injected into their bodies much larger amounts of estrogens than could possibly be absorbed by the skin have not shown any changes toward youthful-looking skins. On the other hand, even the small amounts of estrogens absorbed through the skin can be dangerous to women who may have a tendency toward cancer of the breast or reproductive organs.

Antibiotic Creams

For reasons that are not yet clear, the natural skin oils of some people oxidize rapidly on contact with air and form a fatty, cheeselike substance that plugs the pores. Dust collects in the clogged pores, forming blackheads. Also, certain kinds of bacteria thrive in the fatty substance and cause infections that show up as pimples or boils. This condition is called acne. The exact cause of acne is not known. Sometimes improper diet seems to be the cause, since change in diet clears up the condition. Also, there is no doubt that emotional factors play a part in some cases and hormonal imbalance in others. The cosmetics industry decided that if bacteria play a part in acne, then killing them will cure the disease. A result of this thinking is antibiotic skin cream. This provides a partial relief in many cases, but daily use of antibiotic skin cream carries with it the danger of building up a resistance to the antibiotics. Then, in an emergency, such as a wound or a massive bacterial invasion of the body, antibiotics will be useless.

Shampoos

Healthy hair has a certain amount of oil that keeps it soft and lustrous. Some people have too much oil, some too little, but cosmetics advertising has made almost everyone worry about the amount of oil in her or his hair.

Shampoos are made for both dry hair and oily hair. Those for dry hair contain a moderate amount of soap and/or detergent, oil, and glycerine. The oily-hair shampoos have more detergent and may not have any oil. Either kind of shampoo provides a temporary relief from the dry or oily hair condition. To cure such conditions, medical advice on diet and other factors is necessary.

A current gimmick for shampoos is "protein," which, it is claimed, will thicken thin hair, giving it body, so that it will look fluffy. The protein-like substance in the shampoo is not very soluble in water and sticks to the hair. While it does make hair look thicker, its gluelike properties catch dust at a rate that makes shampooing necessary more frequently than if the protein shampoo were not used—a good situation for the shampoo manufacturers.

Curl and Wave

When the current style calls for curled or wavy hair, the cosmetics industry is ready with a number of curl- and wave-set lotions. These contain chemicals such as thioglyceride, which is a skin irritant. This chemical and others have frequently caused serious skin burns. More important, the setting lotions are often splashed or dripped into the eyes where they cause damaging burns. The *Journal of the American Medical Association* reported a case of a 53-year-old woman who got some wave-set lotion into her ear. The corrosive action of the lotion pierced the woman's eardrum, causing partial deafness.

Hair Dyes

Endless advertising campaigns urge both men and women to change the color of their hair for a variety of reasons. Gray hair is considered to be an especial anathema.

The dyes in hair-coloring preparations are usually coal-tar products—aniline dyes, such as the aminophenols and paradiaminobenzenes. Medical investigation has found many poisonings each year from exposure to such dyes. The kidneys and liver are the organs affected. Coal-tar dyes have long been considered carcinogenic.

Some hair colorings contain fine metallic dust that has been found to cause severe irritation of the nasal passages, throat, and lungs. In some cases the irritation has been so severe that the tissues of the respiratory tract swelled and blocked breathing, making tracheotomies necessary.

Hair Sprays

After hair has been set by wave or curl lotions, it may be kept in place by hair sprays. These are made up of a synthetic resin (polyvinylpyrolidone), dissolved in ethyl alcohol or another solvent. This resin may be fortified by gum arabic or shellac. Perfume and possibly lanolin are added. This mixture is sprayed in a fine mist from an aerosol can, and it is almost impossible to use the spray and not breathe in some of the mist. The resin, lodging in the respiratory tract and the lungs, is not broken down and excreted from the body by the normal metabolic processes. A British doctor found hair-spray type resins intact in liver, lungs, and spleen.

Dentifrices

One of the most advertised cosmetic preparations is toothpaste. The ads claim that toothpaste can do a number of desirable things for the user. It can keep him from having cavities (caries), keep his teeth white or whiten them if they have become discolored, and sweeten his breath.

Tooth decay, which produces caries, is caused by a species of bacterium that thrives on food particles—mainly sugars—which adhere to the teeth. The bacteria produce an acid that dissolves the enamel and dentine of which teeth are made. Toothpastes contain alkaline substances that neutralize the acid, and this is the one useful thing that dentifrices do. Dental experts have long recommended sodium bicarbonate, or baking soda, as an efficient mouth acid neutralizer—and it is much cheaper than toothpaste.

Neutralizing mouth acid is one step in preventing tooth decay; the other is to get rid of food particles that adhere to teeth. This can be accomplished by gentle brushing with a toothbrush. This is the most important step, and if it is done carefully and thoroughly—and the loosened particles are rinsed away with water—no dentifrice is needed. However, it is wise to back up the tooth brushing with a paste of baking soda and water used on the toothbrush in place of toothpaste.

Teeth become discolored for more than one reason. The bacteria which cause decay secrete a very tough gluelike substance that makes food particles adhere to the teeth. Teeth that are not properly brushed will have a layer of food and bacteria accumulate upon them, and the teeth take on a yellowish or brownish color. The best way to prevent this kind of discoloration is to keep the bacteria and food off the surface of the teeth by thorough brushing after each meal and at night before sleeping. Toothpastes contain abrasives which scour away the layer of food and bacteria, but these abrasives also wear away the enamel. Continued brushing with abrasive toothpastes can wear the enamel so thin that the darker dentine beneath shows. This gives the teeth a brownish color, defeating the purpose of toothpaste.

Some dentifrices contain bleaches which may whiten the

teeth but also dissolve the enamel. So, again, the purpose of the tooth "whitener" is eventually defeated.

As for sweetening the breath, a perfumed toothpaste will temporarily give your breath the odor of the perfume for the short time during which it is being dissolved and swallowed. Unpleasant breath comes from decaying teeth, from food left in the interstices of the teeth, or from a throat, lung, or stomach condition. The perfume in a toothpaste cannot get rid of these sources of bad breath, but only mask them temporarily.

Deodorants and Antiperspirants

Perspiration is secreted from two kinds of skin glands, the eccrine and apocrine sweat glands. The *eccrine sweat* glands are found over most of the body. They produce perspiration that is usually odorless. The *apocrine sweat* glands are located in the armpits and the genital region. The sweat they produce is of itself slightly odorous, but the hair follicles of these parts of the body harbor bacteria that work on the substances in apocrine perspiration and create additional odor. Civilized (or at least industrial-cultured) man considers perspiration odor to be obnoxious, so cosmetics manufacturers have created deodorants and antiperspirants to get rid of the odor and launched an advertising campaign (also obnoxious) to reinforce man's fear of his own odors.

Deodorants contain substances that attack the odor-producing bacteria and perfumes that mask the odor. One widely used bacteria-killer is hexachlorophene. In 1972, this chemical was banned for use in hospitals as a bactericidal cleaner and a body wash. Also, it was banned from infant preparations such as salves, lotions, and powders. Although evidence had been mounting for half a dozen years on the harmful effects of this bactericidal chemical, no action was taken until an extra large amount of hexachlorophene was accidently put into a batch of baby powder and killed 36(!) French infants. Finally, authorities became alarmed and banned the chemical.

The amount of hexachlorophene in a daily dose of deodor- ant is small, but the question arises (as always when dealing with small amounts of dangerous substances taken into the body), is the effect of the daily dose cumulative? This is a seri- ous question because hexachlorophene causes brain and cen- tral nervous system damage.

There *are* harmless deodorants. These are creams that con- tain fuller's earth, a very finely divided clay. The fuller's earth does not kill bacteria, but it soaks up and holds perspiration. It must be washed off each day.

Antiperspirants actually stop perspiration for a time. They contain chemicals that cause a slight irritation of the skin that swells the openings of the sweat glands and blocks the excre- tion of perspiration. Unfortunately, this can result in more seri- ous irritation and even infection if staphylococcus bacteria which flourish in perspiration happen to be in the blocked sweat glands. Simply blocking sweat glands defeats nature's purpose of secreting waste products in the perspiration.

Lipsticks

Almost all women who wear lipstick must renew it several times a day because they inadvertently lick it off when talking and eating. In other words, lipstick is actually eaten. Because of this, lipstick should be treated in FDA regulations as food. It is not. The dyes that go into lipstick are not as strictly regu- lated as those that go into food—and the regulations on food are certainly not strict. The FDA's 1960 Color Amendment to the Food, Drug, and Cosmetic Act set temporary tolerances of 6 per cent by weight for 11 coal-tar colors used in lipstick. It is hard to understand the thinking behind this regulation, for two reasons: first, it allows a higher percentage of coal-tar color than is allowed in foods, even though lipstick enters the body in the same way as food; and second, this same regulation pro- hibits coal-tar colors in eye make-up cosmetics because they *might* enter the body, but allows them in lipstick where they are sure to enter the body.

The cosmetics industry tries to justify the use of the dangerous colors by pointing out that there is no case of anyone being poisoned by lipstick. But how many doctors seeing a case of the kind of blood or liver damage caused by coal-tar products would suspect lipstick? As long as it is an established fact that coal-tar colors can be dangerous to health, and that their effect is cumulative, there is no safe amount that can be used in lipstick.

Drugs

Pain-killers, laxatives, tonics, and many other nonprescription drugs are either harmful or useless, as are literally dozens of medicines prescribed by doctors.

Aspirin

Probably the most widely used drug is aspirin. Television and radio commercials exhort Americans to reach for an aspirin whenever they have any kind of ache or pain. Adults can buy aspirin pure or in combination with several other drugs, and children have their own flavored aspirin (and the flavoring of this drug has resulted in the deaths of a number of children who mistook the good-tasting pills for candy). When properly used, aspirin is a valuable pain reliever, but thanks to greedy drug manufacturers whose commercials push the use of aspirin without telling of its dangers, literally thousands of Americans are poisoned in some degree by this drug. In New York City alone, more than 800 persons were accidently poisoned by aspirins in one year—11 per cent of all poisonings in that period. A drug control center in one southwestern state reported 30 cases of aspirin poisoning out of 88 poisoning cases in one month. In Knoxville, Tennessee, a poison control center reported between 40 and 50 cases in one month. Half these were due to parents giving their children overdoses.

The number of abnormal bodily reactions to aspirin is high. Bruce's *Materia Medica*, a standard textbook on medicines, says of aspirin: "Salicylic acid [aspirin] is rapidly absorbed [into the bloodstream] and circulates as sodium salicylate. . . . A moderate dose causes a more rapid heartbeat, a rise in blood pressure, flushing and warmth of the surface, perspiration, fullness in the head, tinnitus [ringing of the ears], deafness, impairment of vision, and possibly a slight rise in temperature. Larger doses may cause delirium, especially with visual hallucinations; respiration is disturbed; the heart is slowed and weakened; the vessels are relaxed and the blood pressure falls; and perspiration is increased. . . . Occasionally, it induces blood or albumin in the urine."

A further list of damaging reactions was given, more than 30 years ago, by the *Journal of the American Medical Association*: "Many reports have appeared on the adverse effects which may follow its unwise use. These have included depression of the heart, habit formation, miscarriage in pregnancy; also, idiosyncrasy [allergic reaction], causing such alarming symptoms as urticaria [hives], pruritis [itching], erythema [redness of the skin], and generalized angoneurotic edema [collection of fluid in the casing of blood vessels and nerves] . . . even ulceration and gangrene have been attributed to its use." Since that report was written, it has been proved that aspirin can cause ulcers of the digestive tract. Also, several different kinds of upset of the endocrine system have been traced to aspirin.

Since irritation of the stomach wall can be caused by bits of aspirin tablets that do not dissolve quickly, the aspirin manufacturers came up with buffered aspirin which, they claimed, dissolved many times as fast as ordinary aspirin. This claim is still used in aspirin advertising despite the findings a dozen years ago by researchers at the University of Buffalo School of Pharmacy that, although buffered aspirin tablets do dissolve faster than plain aspirin, they take longer to disintegrate before dissolving. Thus, there is no advantage in buffered aspirin.

Boric Acid

Boric acid has long been a common item in home medicine cabinets. It was believed to have mild germ-killing properties when dissolved in water and used as a lotion. Boric acid was an ingredient of baby powders (and is still found in some) because its alleged germicidal action would kill bacteria which might be responsible for infants' rashes. Boric acid dissolved in water has also been long recommended as an eyewash.

In the 1960's, a hospital in a northeastern state accidently labeled a bottle of boric acid "dextrose." The acid was then used in the feeding formula of 20 infants. Within 36 hours, all died of severe irritation to the central nervous system. This terrible accident should have been enough to cause authorities to require boric acid to be labeled a poison and its sale to be by prescription only. However, it can still be purchased without prescription in drugstores and supermarkets.

One reason that boric acid is not considered a poison is that it is for external use only. This simply does not take into consideration the numerous cases of infant death caused by dusting with boric acid powder. In 1951, the *American Journal of Diseases of Children* reported a case in which a father put 9 ounces of boric acid on the diapers of his 9-month-old daughter. She died 26 hours later of severe damages of the intestinal tract. The *Journal* said, "Boric acid and sodium borate are sufficiently poisonous to cause severe symptoms and death *when used in amounts commonly considered to be harmless.*" [Emphasis ours] Dr. Harold Abramson, writing in *Pediatrics*, reported another case of infant death due to the use of boric acid on a diaper. Then he wrote, "Boric acid is not a mild and harmless drug. It is quickly absorbed into the body and, in proper amounts, may readily cause toxicity and death."

Furthermore, there are situations in which boric acid may be introduced directly into an infant's mouth. Some popular books on infant care recommend washing nursing-bottle nipples with boric acid. And an infant died after nursing from his mother's breast which had been washed with boric acid.

The medical profession is now aware of the dangers of boric acid and it is being left out of lotions, ointments, and powders. Investigation has shown that boric acid has very little germ-killing power. It is time, then, that the FDA faced the fact that boric acid is a poison and acted to protect the non-medically-trained person who may use the drug with tragic consequences to his family.

Laxatives

Laxatives are probably used as commonly as aspirin. Some users take laxatives every day for most of their lives. There are two main reasons for taking laxatives, both based on false beliefs. One reason—which is plugged in laxative manufacturers' advertising—is that one must be "regular"; that is, must have a daily bowel movement. There is no medical evidence for this. Nature will take care of the elimination of waste matter from the body. This usually happens at daily intervals, but it is not necessary that it should. If conditions, such as dehydration, cause the skipping of bowel movements on one, two, three, or more days, it is nothing to worry about. Nature will eventually cause the intestines to get rid of the accumulated waste matter. If constipation is really caused by a condition that requires that the bowels be cleared, the condition will cause other symptoms besides the constipation. Then, of course, medical help should be sought. In any case, lack of regularity is not a reason for taking a laxative.

A second reason for the continued consumption of laxatives is the belief that the waste matter in the intestine is poisonous and must be eliminated from the body as soon as possible. Waste matter is not poisonous. It is made up of undigested food, broken down blood cells, and other body debris. The toxins that do occur in the body are taken into the intestine for elimination, but this is a one-way process—the toxins go into the intestine; they cannot go out again into the body. In cases of constipation of long duration, toxins may cause difficulty, not because the poisons enter the body from the intestine, but because the accumulation makes it difficult for the body's detoxifying mechanisms to collect more body poisons in the intestine. This happens only in extreme cases.

Some people who are not regular users of laxatives nonetheless are quick to take one when they feel any discomfort in the region of the stomach or bowels. A feeling of being bloated or a pain in the stomach area sends these users to the medicine cabinet for a laxative. This can be dangerous. Appendicitis begins with a pain in the right side just under the ribs. If a laxative is taken because of this pain, it may cause the appendix to rupture, resulting in a serious bloodstream infection. This, we might add, is not uncommon among laxative users.

An appalling number of children have been found to take laxatives—which they of all people certainly do not need—just because their parents take them regularly, or because the laxative looks like chewing gum or chocolate. A child should never be allowed to take a laxative, except under a doctor's orders.

The long-continued use of laxatives eventually damages the normal mechanism of elimination. As a result, the user becomes entirely dependent on drug-induced bowel movements, a condition that can only be cured under medical supervision.

Weight Reducers

Weight-reducing drugs are another product upon which Americans throw away much money and one that too often brings on medical problems. A slim figure for men and women is considered to be very desirable and is sought both by reducing diets and drugs. Losing weight via a reducing diet is slow and difficult; it requires considerable will power to eat only the diet foods. So, a pill that would enable one to eat almost what he pleased in the quantities he pleased, naturally would appeal to those struggling with diets. The drug industry obliged with pills that were alleged to give dieters their wish. But in the more than 15 years since the introduction of reducing pills, they have been shown, time after time, to be worthless or harmful. Nevertheless, the promotion and sale of reducing drugs goes on. The trade publication *Chemical Week* summarized a congressional hearing on weight-reducing drugs by saying that "the pills just don't do the job and overweight consumers are wasting the money they spend on them."

In the same hearing, Dr. Peter Farago, deputy medical director for the FDA, testified (according to the *New York Times*) that one reducing drug, phenylpropanolamine, might have an effect on reducing the appetite if the dosage found in reducing pills were doubled. But doubling the dose might cause heart palpitations, insomnia, and high blood pressure. The problem posed by effective dosages being harmful seems to apply to all reducing drugs.

One kind of reducing preparation is the bulk-producer. This is a liquid which gives a feeling of bulk in the stomach and thereby ends hunger spasms. The danger in this kind of drug is that the person using it will try to substitute it for food, which may result in malnutrition.

Those who believe that they can take off weight quickly with reducing drugs should heed the advice of one health authority: "No easy way is safe; no safe way is easy."

Disastrous Prescription Drugs

The drugs we have been discussing are nonprescription drugs, and it is understandable that the uninformed laymen might harm himself by their misuse. Yet every year there are hundreds of deaths and permanent cripplings due to the prescription of harmful drugs by physicians. These drugs are sold to doctors by criminally irresponsible individuals in drug manufacturing companies.

One tragic example concerns the drug known as MER/29. In 1959, an employee of the William S. Merrell Company estimated that there was a huge potential profit for the drug manufacturer who put on the market a drug that would maintain normal cholesterol levels in the blood. Cholesterol is a substance, produced mainly by the liver, which is found normally in the bloodstream. Statistics seem to indicate that persons with higher-than-normal levels of cholesterol in their blood will develop hardening of the arteries (atherosclerosis) which leads to high blood pressure (hypertension), stroke, and heart disease. The FDA said in December 1959, that a "causal relationship between blood cholesterol levels and [heart and artery] diseases has not been proven." Yet, many physicians believed that the statistics pointed to such a relationship. The people at Merrell estimated that if everyone over 35 took one anticholesterol tablet a day, the company would do a $4,250,000,000 business in this one drug alone. Even if only one-fourth of those over 35 used the drug regularly, the profits would still be fantastic.

A Merrell chemist named Frank Palopoli had been working on an anticholesterol drug that now seemed marketable. In July 1959, Merrell filed with the FDA a New Drug Application for a substance they called MER/29. The 285-page application included a statement that "full reports of all investigations have been made to show whether or not the drug is safe for use." The reports included a description of the test work on laboratory animals and clinical trials of the drug on 116 patients at seven medical centers.

On April 9, 1960, the FDA made the New Drug Application effective, despite strong misgivings by some FDA investigators. Merrell immediately launched a multimillion dollar advertising campaign aimed at doctors. MER/29 was termed by the advertising as "the first safe agent to inhibit body-produced cholesterol." So-called detail men, actually drug salesmen, visited physicians' offices pushing MER/29. The drug company's 1961

Annual Report stated that MER/29 was the nation's "leading anticholesterol drug," and that it was the company's "largest-selling" prescription drug.

Meanwhile, reports of serious side-effects of MER/29 were piling up. Some patients had developed ichthyosis (fishlike condition), a painful scaly skin malady, and began to lose their hair. Other patients developed cataracts, a disease in which the lens of the eye becomes permanently clouded, resulting in blindness. Ceasing to take the drug ended the skin disease and began a regrowth of hair. Cataract blindness, however, could be treated only by surgical removal of the opaque lens and the use of special thick eyeglasses.

This increasing evidence that MER/29 was toxic disturbed the FDA, and several staff members wanted Merrell to withdraw the drug. Merrell, of course, did not want to lose its chief moneymaker. It resisted suggestions that the drug be taken off the market.

One evening in February 1962, Thomas Rice, a Cincinnati inspector for the FDA, was riding in a car pool with Carson Jordan, husband of a former employee at Merrell. Jordan mentioned that his wife had worked in Merrell's toxicologypathology laboratory and that she had once been told to falsify a chart depicting research involving MER/29. Rice interviewed Mrs. Jordan and then informed the FDA in Washington. About a month and a half later, Rice and two medical officers of the FDA visited Merrell's laboratories armed with a certificate of inspection. Within two days they found that information given to the FDA in the New Drug Application had been falsified. The next day, Merrell informed the FDA that it was taking MER/29 off the market.

In a speech given to an American Bar Association group, Deputy Food and Drug Commissioner John L. Harvey admitted that "in retrospect, it is apparent that the drug should not have gone on the market in the first place." This admission was slightly comforting to the reformers who planned on getting further bans againsts drugs, but not much use to those already blinded by MER/29.

The government took legal action against the William S. Merrell Company. The net result of this action was a fine of $88,000 and sentences of six months probation against the three Merrell employees most closely connected with and responsible for falsifying the scientific data. In civil suits, Merrell paid between $45 and $55 million to those harmed by MER/29.

Kevadon-Thalidomide—Merrell Again

A month before Merrell withdrew MER/29 from the market, it had withdrawn Kevadon, a sleep-inducing compound, from the Canadian market and from about 1,000 American physicians who were about to use it in clinical investigation programs.

Kevadon was Merrell's name for Thalidomide, which had been developed by a West German pharmaceutical company, Chemie Grünenthal. This compound, used in sleeping pills, induced a gentle slumber without the undesirable effects of barbiturate-based drugs. Thalidomide soon became West Germany's most popular sleep-inducing drug. It was even put into a liquid form for children and recommended for pregnant women who suffered from morning sickness.

Six years later, the William S. Merrell Company obtained from the German firm the rights to manufacture and market the drug in the U.S. and Canada. Merrell geared up a very high-pressure sales campaign while its New Drug Application was pending approval at the FDA. Detail men fanned out to get advance orders for Kevadon.

At the FDA the New Drug Application was given to Dr. Frances Kelsey. She shared an office with Dr. John Nestor, who at the time was involved with Merrell concerning MER/29. When Merrell's liaison people in Washington realized that Dr. Kelsey was not going to approve Kevadon quickly, they feared her approval might not meet the date, March 6, 1961, that Merrell had set for sales release of the drug. Officers of the company put unremitting pressure on her, but she made it clear that she would not be rushed.

Dr. Kelsey wrote a detailed letter to Merrell stating why she thought the company's application was incomplete and did not adequately demonstrate safety. She made a brilliant deduction: Kevadon induced sleep in human beings but not in test animals; therefore, although the drug might be safe for animals, it was not necessarily safe for human beings. She asked the company to submit more information on the pharmacological properties of the drug and also on human case histories of use of Kevadon. The company replied with the requested information. Dr. Kelsey asked her husband, who was a physician-pharmacologist, to analyze Merrell's data. He found that it was an "interesting collection of meaningless pseudoscientific jargon apparently intended to impress chemically unsophisticated readers." Also, he pointed out that the company had made a statement that violated "an elementary concept of pharmacy" and he did not "believe this to be honest incompetence."

While Merrell was continuing to put pressure on Dr. Kelsey, she came across a letter, in the *British Medical Journal* in which a physician reported that four of his patients who had taken Thalidomide experienced abnormal numbing and tingling of their hands and feet. A second letter, from the German drug firm, said there were other reports of the same symptoms which could be forerunners of a serious malady, peripheral neuritis. For this reason the company was including a warning in their literature saying that if the symptoms appeared, use of the drug should be discontinued.

Dr. Kelsey wondered what might be the effect of the drug on a fetus exposed to it for a long time. When she informed Merrell of this, they tried to pooh-pooh the letters in the British journal, pointing out that the British were "merely adding a warning," not banning the drug. Two company officials flew to Europe to study the peripheral neuritis reports. Upon returning, they called the neuritis a minor drawback which was outweighed by Kevadon's advantages over barbiturates. Dr. Kelsey felt that the men were "at no time being wholly frank," and she was suspicious of their "failure to notify us of the British reports of toxicity."

The drug company continued to pressure Dr. Kelsey, but she would not be moved. Bits of evidence against the drug continued to appear. Merrell moved its hoped-for marketing date up to the middle of November 1961, but by that date, Dr. Kelsey was still not convinced that Kevadon was safe.

Meanwhile, the Canadian Food and Drug Directorate had approved Merrell's application to market Kevadon, and the drug was sold widely in Canada.

On November 29, Merrell received a cablegram from Chemie Grünenthal saying that Thalidomide had been removed from the market because it was suspected of causing birth defects. Merrell did not seem to think that this information was serious enough to warrant withdrawal of Kevadon from Canada. But they did send every physician in Canada a letter in which they warned that "Kevadon should not be administered to pre-menopausal women who may become pregnant."

Despite all the evidence against Thalidomide, Merrell did not withdraw its New Drug Application. An official of the company wrote to Canadian physicians that there was "still no positive proof of a causal relationship between the use of Thalidomide during pregnancy and malformations in the newborn." The official also stated, almost idiotically, that it was encouraging to note that studies on pregnant rats had not shown a single malformation in more than 1,100 offspring of the Thalidomide-treated animals. This latter statement simply proved Dr. Kelsey's fear that since Thalidomide did not induce sleep in test animals, they might not develop the same side effects as human beings. Later tests showed that Thalidomide did cause birth defects in pregnant rabbits. (This fact points to the tragic mischance that rats instead of rabbits were chosen as the test animals.)

In its February 23, 1962, issue, *Time* magazine told the heart-rending story of Thalidomide in West Germany. It revealed that thousands of babies had been born deformed. The more "fortunate" infants were born without hands or legs or with flipper-like appendages where their limbs should have been. The worst were inhumanly shapeless lumps of flesh.

Time's story revealed that Kevadon was still being sold in Canada. Amid the storm of outrage and anxiety that arose, the chief of Canada's Food and Drug Directorate said that Kevadon did not have to be withdrawn because Canada "has no cases yet" and the drug's connection with birth deformities was not causal, but "only statistical." Newsmen were told by an FDD spokesman that no swift action was necessary and that they "shouldn't jump off the deep end." A week later, officials of the FDD changed their minds and asked Merrell to withdraw Kevadon-Thalidomide.

Dr. Kelsey's intelligence and courage saved the women of the United States from living the tragic nightmare of their German sisters. On August 7, 1962, President Kennedy awarded her the Distinguished Federal Civilian Service Award "for her high ability and steadfast confidence in her professional decision."

For some months after both MER/29 and Kevadon were withdrawn from the market, Merrell officials kept putting out, to physicians and any others they could reach, mendacious statements such as one saying that "Merrell has vigorously pursued a course that is in the best interest of the public welfare, both in terms of human safety and scientific and medical research."

The stories of MER/29 and Kevadon are frightening because they illustrate that no one can be certain that his doctor is not prescribing a drug which can do terrible damage instead of accomplishing its intended cure.

How can this happen? First, physicians are overwhelmingly busy and cannot keep up with the flood of medical literature. This leaves them unaware of information that might alert them to the dangers of a drug they are prescribing. Also, while most doctors know enough not to believe detail men, too many doctors believe the drug company's literature. And many have too much faith in the drug manufacturers' scientists, believing that the rigors of science preclude dishonesty on the part of pharmaceutical researchers.

More important is the fact that physicians are offered new drugs that can do the damage done by MER/29 and Thalidomide. So, the main responsibility seems to lie with a system that relies on the good faith of drug manufacturers whose overwhelming concern is profit. The concern for money results in corrupted research scientists and, in turn, dangerous drugs. What is more, it is far too easy, as Congressman Benjamin S. Rosenthal of New York pointed out, for lawyers, physicians, and research scientists to slip in and out of government, going from positions in regulatory agencies to positions in drug manufacturing firms and back again. In such cases, the public interest is not likely to be the official's main concern.

Ralph Adam Fine, a Department of Justice Attorney and author of an excellent book detailing the MER/29 and Thalidomide stories, set forth two conditions that could go a long way toward diminishing the abuses of the drug industry. They are:

1. New drugs . . . must be thoroughly tested before being released for general sale (whether by prescription or over the counter). This testing should be under the strict direct supervision of either the government or an independent group *with no financial stake in the results.* [Italics ours.]

2. The totality of a drug company's experience with a drug (excluding, of course, bona fide trade secrets) must be made

available to any interested person. A physician cannot properly balance the risks of a certain treatment against its expected benefits unless he has all the information. "Puffing," the business euphemism for fraudulent advertising, "must not be permitted."

Our Sad State of Health

The United States is the wealthiest nation and its citizens are the healthiest people in the world. True or false? Half true. We *are* the wealthiest nation, but according to the United Nations World Health Organization, the people of the United States are ranked twelfth in health. Our supermarkets burst with food and the variety of foods exceeds that found in any other nation, yet we are not a healthy people. The reason for this shouldn't be hard to find.

We have seen that we American consumers face a daily body-polluting threat to our health from the use of toxic pesticides and the overuse of chemical fertilizers. The same kind of threat comes from the thousands of additives in our foods. Still further threats to health come from the cosmetics and drugs that have become a part of our lives.

In addition to the harmful substances in our food, we are appallingly ignorant of the simplest knowledge of nutrition. We eat the wrong kinds of foods, too little or too much, and prepare the food poorly.

Life Expectancy in the United States

One of the things various health agencies point to with pride is the fact that the average American has a life expectancy of approximately 70 years. This is nearly double that of his ancestor of a century ago, who could look forward to only 36 years. But if we look carefully at this statistic it becomes less impressive. The life expectancy of a people is an average figure and is lowered by deaths in early years. A century ago, lack of obstetrical care, meager knowledge of infants' diseases, and mortal gastrointestinal diseases from impure milk resulted in a high death rate among infants. Scarlet fever, diphtheria, and tuberculosis accounted for many deaths in early childhood. It was this high mortality rate in infancy and childhood that pulled down the life-expectancy average to the frighteningly low 36 years. However, the individual 19th century American who survived to the age of 40 had a further life expectancy of only two years less than his descendant of today. And our ancestors who reached 60 could expect to continue living longer than today's 60-year-olds. In other words, we have increased our life expectancy through the excellent work done by the medical profession in delivering more healthy babies and pulling them through early childhood.

That we have been able to increase a mature individual's life span by only two years in a century—100 years of amazing advances in surgical techniques, public health measures, and drugs that pull seriously ill persons away from death's door— points to a great failure in keeping the general health of the whole population on a high level. Any doubt that something is very wrong with this nation's health should be dispelled by the fact that our life expectancy is *going down*. In 1961, it reached a high of 70.2 years. Two years later, it was down to 70, and in 1968, had dropped to 69.8 years. During the years the life expectancy was dropping, the death rate from degenerative diseases—heart disease, kidney disease, gastrointestinal ulcers— was rising. The American male actually has a poor life expectancy when compared to that of the American women. A man's life expectancy, in 1969, was 66.8 years, while a woman's was 73.7. And the American male makes a poor showing when compared to males of other countries. In Sweden, a man could expect to live 71.6 years, and those of 25 other countries also could expect to live longer than the average American man.

Other pieces of evidence that there is something very wrong with the American health scene are:

The American Heart Association reports that the United States leads the world in deaths from heart disease.

Twenty-three countries have a lower infant mortality rate than we do.

Rejection of armed forces draftees for physical and mental deficiencies is well above the 40 per cent rate.

An examination of 10,000 highly placed business executives found only one in ten to have normal health.

Over a ten-year period, the proportion of patients admitted to hospitals rose five times faster than the population increased.

One family in seven has a member who undergoes surgery in a given year.

These depressing statistics could be expanded greatly, but there would be no point in doing so. Our purpose has been to make it clear that the state of health of the population of the United States is deplorable. We have shown in an earlier part of this book, providing considerable detail, that the American consumer daily ingests a whole host of poisons which certainly contribute to the low level of health. Let us now see in detail what are the nutritional deficiencies in our national diet.

Affluence and Malnutrition

Americans eat more food per individual than any other people. Yet we have a high and increasing percentage of deficiency diseases. This can only mean that we are stuffing ourselves with food and starving at the same time. The same deficiency diseases that plague overweight Americans are found in parts of the world where people simply do not have enough to eat and so do not get sufficient nutrients to be healthy. Therefore, Americans must be eating large quantities of foods that lack the nutrients necessary for good health. More than two decades of research have shown that Americans suffer from a kind of malnutrition that comes not from lack of calories, but from diets that are deficient in protein, vitamins, and minerals.

In 1953, *Newsweek* carried an article on one group of malnourished Americans: teenagers. "American teenagers," the article said, "even those of high income families, are gravely undernourished. A well-known nutrition authority has come to this conclusion after a ten-year study of 2,536 boys and girls between the ages of 13 and 20 years. The following findings were revealed:

"1. Only about 25 per cent of the boys and girls were eating sufficient energy-making foods to keep the body machinery running efficiently.

"2. Nearly half of the girls (a few less of the boys) lacked the proper amount of protein foods necessary to build and repair body tissues.

"3. Both boys and girls showed a shortage of calcium and phosphorus, vital for good teeth and bones, and of iron—related to good red blood and needed to prevent anemia.

"4. Forty-nine per cent of the boys and 48 per cent of the girls suffered from "nutritional nerves"—twitching of the face, nail-biting and restlessness. (This is usually indicative of a lack of the Vitamin B complex.)

"5. There was a serious vitamin shortage, including vitamins A, B, and C in both boys' and girls' diets.

"6. Only seven girls and twelve boys of the 2,536 examined had perfect teeth. (Tooth decay is evidence of dietary deficiencies.)

"7. Eighteen per cent of the girls and 19 per cent of the boys were underweight.

"8. Eye trouble, caused by poor diet, particularly a lack of vitamin A, was evident in more than three-quarters of the adolescents examined.

"9. Poor complexions, acne, and rough skin were the rule, with girls making a worse showing than the boys."

The foregoing situation is borne out by other studies. One, which included 59,000 boys and girls in 38 states, revealed that teenage malnutrition is nationwide. Studies show that the average child is properly nourished only up to the age of two; after that, his diet declines until it reaches a low in his teens.

Dr. H. Curtis Wood, Jr., obstetrician, gynecologist, and nutrition consultant, writes in his book, *Overfed but Undernourished*, "Young people have an amazing ability to adjust and adapt to unbelievably deficient diets and yet feel fairly well. Because of this, they do not understand that while they may be able to get away with living on hamburgers, potato chips and soda pop without apparent disastrous results for some years, it will eventually catch up with them in one way or another."

We suggest that one of the most needed courses of instruction in our public schools is the subject of nutrition. One hour a week for a few years would pay invaluable health dividends for the rest of a student's life.

The nutritional situation among adults is little better than among teenagers. The Department of Agriculture made a nutritional survey in 1965 and announced its results in 1968. Seventy-five hundred households were surveyed and believed to be representative of national economic and geographic groups. One finding was that only 50 per cent of all households had diets that were considered nutritious. Twenty per cent subsist on wholly inadequate diets. In a similar survey done in 1955, 15 per cent of American households had inadequate diets. Thus, we are becoming more and more poorly fed. Although the largest group of the ill nourished—36 per cent— was from families with incomes under $3,000 per year, 9 per cent of upper income families had inadequate diets. Poor nutrition, then, is not limited to poor people, but is found even among the affluent. Former Secretary of Agriculture Orville Freeman commented on his department's survey: "We must conclude that many Americans are making a poor choice, nutritionally, of our food abundance and that to a large extent income does not determine good nutrition."

Except for the lowest income group whose members cannot afford enough nourishing foods, obtaining a nutritious diet is simply a matter of knowledge and choice—knowing what and how much to eat and choosing to act on this knowledge. From the indication of the statistics, Americans don't know what a nourishing diet is or they don't care, or both.

It seems reasonable that if most people understood the effects of poor nutrition, they probably would make it their business to eat a nourishing diet. On the other hand, this may not be true. Dr. Wood states that the "medical establishment has an extraordinary antipathy to the idea that nutrition is important for good health, quite inexplicable in view of the various dietary diseases described in any medical textbook." He goes on to say that doctors are aware of the more serious deficiency diseases such as pellagra, beriberi, scurvy, and xerothalmia, but they do not seem to recognize the symptoms of lesser nutritional deficiencies such as bleeding gums and easy bruising, which are caused by vitamin C deficiency.

Vitamin Deficiencies and Health

Xerothalmia is a dry, thickened condition of the eyeball, which can lead to blindness. It is common in countries where the diet is lacking in fresh fruits and vegetables. The precise ingredient lacking in such a diet is vitamin A. Also caused by vitamin A deficiency is night blindness. Despite the abundance of fresh produce in the United States, physicians encounter xerothalmia in their patients, and night blindness is not uncommon.

Keratomalacia is a clouding of the cornea, the transparent covering of the pupil of the eye. Extreme clouding of the lens of the eye is known as cataract. Both of these diseases are common in India, where the average diet is nutritionally poor. A missionary doctor tells of his experience which clearly links these eye diseases to vitamin A. He would give Indians suffering from keratomalacia a large injection of vitamin A, and within 24 hours, their blurred vision cleared up almost entirely.

An interesting experiment connecting cataracts with nutrition was performed at Johns Hopkins University and reported in 1970. Thirty rats were given an exclusive diet of yogurt. All 30 developed cataracts. The disease took only $1\frac{1}{2}$ months to develop in the six youngest, and a little longer in the older rats. The experimenters said it was very unusual to have every rat in an experiment develop the same disease. They also said that the rats had been bred from a colony that Johns Hopkins had been keeping for 40 years and "to our knowledge, no rat in the 40-year-old colony . . . ever developed cataracts spontaneously." Thus, the scientists believed, it had to be something in the rats' diet that caused the disease. The experimenters decided that it was one of the components in the milk sugar, lactose, which is part of yogurt. Dr. Wood, who commented on the experiment, pointed out that, instead of being an ingredient of yogurt, the cause could have been some food components that were lacking in the very limited diet.

There is an exciting theory on the role of nutrition in a fairly common eye disease known as detached retina. The retina is the light-sensitive layer of cells that coats the inner eye. Sometimes the retina becomes detached from the inner wall of the eye. A small part may separate or the whole retina may detach, causing blindness in the latter case.

The present treatment for detached retina is surgical. In a very delicate operation, thin needles are inserted into the eye so that their tips are between the separated retina and the tissue behind it. A weak electric current is then sent through the needles. It is hoped that the current will coagulate some of the fluid that fills the eye and thereby glue the retina back in place. Unfortunately, this treatment is not a sure cure.

There are some who believe that a nutritional cure is possible. They are impressed with the role of vitamin C in what is known as "intercellular cement substances." In the absence of these substances, tiny blood vessels break and bleeding occurs. It is possible, then, that in the absence of sufficient vitamin C, the tiny blood vessels behind the retina break and the resulting hemorrhage pushes the retina away from the tissue behind it.

Hearing and Diet

There are more than 20 million deaf persons in the United States—just about one in ten. There are many kinds of deafness, two of which—chronic progressive deafness and tinnitus (ringing in the ears)—may be due to a lack of vitamin A. *Eye, Ear, Nose, and Throat Monthly* reported that two doctors had injected 50,000-unit doses of vitamin A every two weeks into 24 hard-of-hearing patients. After three injections, 16 showed definite improvement in hearing; six out of nine who had tinnitus were greatly relieved. Large doses of the vitamin B-complex also have relieved chronic progressive deafness.

A very serious aural disease is Meniere's syndrome. It is characterized by a loud ringing in the ears and also by nausea, vertigo (dizziness and loss of balance), and tinnitus. A contributor to the *Archives of Otolaryngology* divided sufferers from Meniere's syndrome into three groups and reported:

"All three groups show signs of chronic, severe deficiency of the vitamin B-complex (thiamine, nicotinic acid and riboflavin all being involved). . . . The attacks of vertigo can be controlled by the administration of the appropriate vitamins in suitable dosage and tinnitus can often be considerably relieved with the same regimen. . . . Patients in the age group in which

Meniere's disease commonly arises, forty to sixty years, require a high protein, high vitamin, moderate-to-low carbohydrate and low fat diet. *It is a rarity to find such a diet.* Yet if patients with Meniere's syndrome are to be restored to full health and efficiency and not merely relieved of their attacks, insistence on such a diet is essential."

Nutrition and Teeth

The most prevalent disease in the United States is dental caries, or cavities. A Public Health Service estimate put the number of caries at more than a billion. If all the dentists in the country were to work eight hours a day, seven days a week, on filling caries, they would never catch up with all the cavities that needed filling. While it is possible for an individual to have all his caries filled, simply approaching the problem this way is a losing game. Eventually, his teeth will be a mass of fillings. Obviously, prevention of tooth decay is the best approach. We all are taught in home and school that one way to prevent tooth decay is by keeping the teeth clean. This means brushing them after each meal and before going to sleep. The purpose of this activity is to remove food that clings to the teeth and provides nourishment for the bacteria that cause decay. This care is very important, but alone it will not entirely prevent caries. Dental hygiene must be coupled with a nutritious diet.

A Canadian-born dentist, Dr. Weston A. Price, traveled to 45 countries seeking an answer to the question, "Why do some peoples of the world have good teeth, while those of other peoples are so poor?" He visited the remote regions of Canada and Alaska, examining the teeth of the less civilized Indians. He compared the teeth of the Indians who traded with the white man and had contacts with white man's culture and the teeth of Indians who remained isolated from white civilization. Those who lived away from white civilization had only 0.16

per cent tooth decay, while those who ate white man's food had 21.5 per cent decay. Dr. Price found that the latter group were getting 83 per cent less calcium, 83 per cent less phosphorus, 64 per cent less iron, 76 per cent less copper, 89 per cent less iodine, and much less vitamin A than those with good teeth. To whichever country Dr. Price went, he found the same situation: good diet and good teeth went together. People who ate devitalized processed foods invariably had poor teeth.

Diseases of the gums and the bone in which the teeth are imbedded also are caused by dietary deficiency. If the gums and bone are not healthy, the teeth cannot be healthy. The health of all these structures depends on ingesting sufficient calcium, fluorine, phosphorus, iodine, magnesium, and vitamins A and C. All these substances can be obtained from a diet that includes bone meal, dairy products, fish and fish oils, sea kelp, and citrus fruits.

Since a child's first teeth begin to grow before it is born, the mother must provide her developing child with the necessary nutritive elements by eating the proper foods herself.

Laboratory experiments have demonstrated that fluoride ions can replace hydroxyl and bicarbonate ions on the surface of bones, forming a highly resistant and insoluble substance called fluorapatite. This exchange can take place in the enamel of teeth when the fluoride is ingested in a number of ways: in foods such as bone meal, in drinking water, in toothpaste, or when a fluoride compound is painted on the teeth. The fluorapatite coating that forms on the teeth resists decay. The bacteria that cause decay produce an acid that does the actual eroding of the enamel, but this acid does not successfully attack a fluorapatite surface on a tooth. So the effect of fluoride ingested in one or another way is to cut down the number of dental caries.

Fluorides are now added to the drinking water of perhaps a majority of towns and cities in the United States, most of which report a drop in the tooth decay suffered by their citizens. For reasons we won't discuss here, there is a considerable amount of opposition to the practice of putting fluorides in public drinking water. Most nutritionists oppose it, and most medical and dental associations approve it.

Diet and Skin

Nutritionists and physicians agree that the condition of the skin may reflect an individual's physical and emotional health. A number of skin diseases are known to be due to dietary and emotional factors.

Pellagra is a serious skin disease that once was prevalent in large areas of the southern United States. In these areas, most people's diets were restricted to pork and cornmeal for long periods. The disease begins with lassitude, weakness, loss of appetite, and indigestion. Later, a horrible skin rash on the back and neck, red tongue, ulcerated mouth, diarrhea, and dementia appear. All of these symptoms disappear when the pellagra sufferer is fed a diet that includes beef, eggs, and fresh milk, which contain niacin, a member of the vitamin B-complex and the substance that effects the cure.

Follicular hyperkeratosis is another skin disease caused by nutritional deficiency. In this fairly common disease, the patient has very rough dry skin that is covered with little bumps, making it resemble gooseflesh. In approximately one-third of the cases, the tiny bumps become infected and form little pimples. A diet rich in vitamin A will cure or prevent follicular hyperkeratosis.

Not all skin diseases respond to nutritional therapy. Two of these are the common and very unpleasant acne and psoriasis. However, as a general rule, a seriously inadequate diet results in some kind of diseased skin condition, and this condition can be eliminated by a nutritionally adequate diet.

Diet and Hair

In some ways a hair is like a blade of grass. Both grow from roots through which they take in the substances they need for health and growth. Knowing this fact, you can easily see that what substances a hair takes in depends on what the owner of the hair has in his or her bloodstream (the nourishment enters the hair root through tiny blood vessels). And what is in the bloodstream depends heavily on what a person is eating. There are many hair diseases, and though a direct link between them and diet has not yet been established, it can be demonstrated that diet does have an effect on hair. This is dramatically seen in animals, such as stray cats and dogs, that have been on a starvation diet for a few months. These animals always have coats of dull, thin hair. Taken into a home and fed well, stray cats and dogs invariably develop thick, glossy coats. The role of diet in this change would be hard to deny. Two other proofs that there is a connection between diet and hair condition are seen in the fact that the normally black hair of African children assumes a reddish tint if the child is undernourished, and the black hair of Mexican children turns a yellowish color when they are undernourished. Also, there are cases in which gray hair turned back to its former color when its owner added vitamin B-complex to his diet.

Diet and Arthritis

Arthritis is one of the major crippling diseases. In the United States, more than 13 million persons suffer from it, including 200,000 children under 14, of whom 50,000 are pre-schoolers. Arthritis is an ancient disease; Egyptian mummies show unmistakable evidence of it. The symptoms are severe pain and distortion of the joints, resulting in the disability of the patient. As far as the medical profession is concerned, there is no cure for arthritis. Most doctors treat arthritic patients with pain-killers, mainly aspirin. More sophisticated pain-relieving treatment includes the injection of cortisone and gold salts. However, there have been a sufficient number of dramatic cures of arthritis to contradict categorically the statement that there is no cure. And the cures have been due to diet.

Mr. Karl Barr Lutz, a layman with a knowledge of biochemistry, discovered a dietary arthritis cure by curing himself of the disease. Mr. Lutz went further than a cure; he sought a possible cause. He learned that arthritis is one of the so-called "collagen diseases." Collagen is a connective tissue that takes several forms in the body. One of these is cartilage, which lines the joints of the bones. Since collagen is found in many parts of the body, it is not hard to understand the statement made by the Arthritis and Rheumatism Foundation that "one point needs to be heavily underscored: *the entire body is affected by arthritis*—even though only the joints are inflamed." This was a tipoff that arthritis might respond to dietary treatment.

Seeking the components of such a diet, Mr. Lutz found out several things about collagen. There was the following statement by Dr. Jerome Gross, of Harvard Medical School: "Collagen is probably the most abundant protein in the animal kingdom." Therefore, it seems reasonable that emphasis should be placed on establishing good protein metabolism—good intake and assimilation. This should be basic to the prevention and cure of arthritis.

"Vitamin C," according to Bicknell and Prescott in *The Vitamins in Medicine*, "is directly implicated in the activity of the adrenal cortex." Vitamin C may stimulate secretion of cortisone and other hormones that come from the adrenal glands. Since injection of cortisone provides temporary relief of arthritic inflamation, vitamin C may accomplish the same thing naturally. This vitamin maintains the elasticity of capillary blood vessels. In its absence, the vessels break and blood flows into the surrounding tissue. When these tiny hemorrhages occur in the joints, there is a flareup of arthritis pain.

In a 1943 article in the *Physiological Review*, Mary E. Reid showed that, in the formation of collagen, enough calcium must be present along with the vitamin C and protein.

In 1957, Dr. Hugh Sinclair of the Laboratory of Human Nutrition, Oxford University, stated that unsaturated fats (found in vegetable oils, fish, and some other foods) are needed for strong collagen tissue.

One more thing necessary for proper collagen metabolism is the correct amount of hydrochloric acid in the stomach. The secretion of this acid decreases after the age of 20, so it is common to find a lack of it in older persons, the chief arthritis sufferers.

With the foregoing facts in hand, Mr. Lutz worked out the following nutritional program for the treatment of arthritis.

1) For *improved protein metabolism,* increase the intake of high quality protein and correct the hydrochloric acid secretion in the stomach so that the protein can be properly assimilated.

2) *Increase the intake of vitamin C* and avoid the vitamin C antagonists such as caffeine, inhaled cigarette smoke, and residues from pesticides which are found in most mass-produced foodstuffs.

3) *Increase the intake of calcium.*

4) *Ingest ample amounts of unsaturated fats.*

In addition to the above, the rest of the diet should be well balanced. Supplementary amounts of the other vitamins (besides vitamin C) and minerals (in addition to calcium) should be included. An analysis of stomach fluid can be made to learn of possible lack of hydrochloric acid, and a blood analysis will spot any other nutritional deficiencies.

Osteoporosis

Another common bone disease is osteoporosis, a condition in which bones become demineralized. The bones lose mainly calcium, but also phosphorus and magnesium. The normal passages within the bones enlarge and new spaces form, resulting in fragile bones. This condition is prevalent in persons over 50.

Researchers have found that this disease can be reversed; calcium and other minerals can be redeposited in bones that have lost them. This redeposition can be accomplished in several ways. One medical group gave osteoporosis patients massive doses of calcium salts. Results were excellent. Good results can also be obtained by including a pint of milk in the daily diet of patients. Milk, however, may bring its own problems: kidney, gall stones, or increased cholesterol in the blood. A very satisfactory way of obtaining the needed calcium is in tablet form. The tablets usually are made of calcium lactate or calcium gluconate, with or without vitamin D, which aids in the metabolism of calcium. Eight hundred milligrams per day is the recommended dosage. The Marion Laboratories of Kansas City, Missouri, sell a tablet made from oyster shells, which are composed of calcium carbonate. This compound makes available to the body 40 per cent elemental calcium, which is 27 per cent more than is available from calcium lactate.

Diseases of the Heart and Blood Vessels

Heart and blood vessel diseases cause the deaths of more than one million Americans a year. Degenerative heart disease —angina pectoris, coronary heart disease, chronic myocarditis, and myocardial degeneration—is the chief single cause of death in the United States, especially after the age of 40. These same heart conditions are almost rare in some parts of Europe. One set of statistics notes that in Italy—where the diet includes only half as much fat as in the United States (20 per cent in Italy, 40 per cent in the U.S.)—death from degenerative heart disease between the ages of 40 and 45 is 20 per cent of ours; from 50 to 54, 23 per cent; and from 60 to 64, 24 per cent.

Researchers have been able to produce heart disease in a

number of ways: by feeding laboratory animals diets high in saturated fats; by depriving the animals of vitamin B_6, pyridoxine; and by depriving them of vitamin C.

A clearcut causal relationship between smoking and heart disease has been established. The reason that smoking causes heart disease probably lies in the fact that nicotine, one of the ingredients of tobacco, is a vitamin C antagonist that destroys the vitamin in the body.

Another suspected cause of heart disease is lack of vitamin E. Dr. Wilfred E. Shute, of the Shute Institute, London, Ontario, says that the rate of coronary heart disease first began to increase when steel-roller mills began to remove the wheat germ from flour. The germ is rich in vitamine E. Dr. Shute has successfully treated thousands of heart patients with vitamin E therapy.

High Blood Pressure and Cholesterol

Thanks to much publicity by the American Heart Association, large numbers of Americans know that cholesterol has something to do with high blood pressure and heart disease. A high level of cholesterol in the blood, along with saturated fats, causes atherosclerosis, or hardening of the arteries. When there is a large amount of these two substances in the blood, tiny platelets of fat collect on the walls of the blood vessels, narrowing the passage through which blood can flow. (The thicker the deposit of fatty substance on the arterial walls the "harder" the artery.) As the heart tries to pump the same amount of blood through narrowed arteries as it pumped through wide arteries, two things happen: the pressure of the blood in the blood vessel goes up and the heart has to work harder. High blood pressure may rupture small blood vessels in the brain, and the resulting hemorrhage causes a stroke. A heart which is continually overworked develops enlarged blood vessels that may eventually rupture, causing death.

There is no sure way of avoiding all types of heart disease, but the degenerative kind that results from hardening of the arteries can be greatly slowed, if not altogether avoided, by a diet low in cholesterol and unsaturated fats and high in vitamin E (200 I.U. per day, or more when prescribed by a physician), vitamin C (2000 mg. per day), and vitamin B-complex. Smoking should be avoided because, as we have seen, cigarette smoke contains a vitamin antagonist. There should be a daily intake of calcium from either one pint of milk, three bone meal tablets, or three calcium lactate tablets. Foods containing lecithin and linoleic acid should be in the diet.

The Common Cold

It has been estimated that in the United States in midwinter, thirty million men, women, and children have colds at any given time. Despite considerable research, the cause of the common cold remains unknown. Until very recently, there was nothing to be done about a cold, except to wait for it to "go away." Now, a very efficient cure is known. It consists simply in sufficient daily doses of vitamin C. Dr. Curtis Wood, Jr., says that ascorbic acid (vitamin C) destroys viruses in the blood by oxidizing them. An unknown type of virus may be the cause of colds, so if it is, this fact would account for the effectiveness of vitamin C therapy.

Since vitamin C is rapidly eliminated by the kidneys, it is necessary to take frequent doses in order to keep a high level of the vitamin in the blood. Dr. Linus Pauling, winner of Nobel Prizes in both chemistry and peace, recommends 1000 mg. of vitamin C every hour when you feel a cold coming on. To keep from getting a cold, 3000 mg. per day is recommended. Within these limits, vitamin C is safe, and also inexpensive if one does not buy it as prepared by some of the larger pharmaceutical companies, but rather in supermarkets, cut-rate drugstores or health food stores. The fact that vitamin C is an inexpensive and effective cold remedy is the main reason that its use has been fought by the pharmaceutical industry. And they have reason to worry, since Americans spend more than $500 million on cold "remedies" that do little more than lessen the unpleasant symptoms a bit. If vitamin C therapy were to become widely used, most of the drug industry's $500 million would be lost.

Lung Cancer

One of the tragic and unnecessary scourges of life in the United States is lung cancer caused by smoking cigarettes. Smoking is not the only cause of lung cancer, but it is a major cause and a needless one.

By the early 1960's, the evidence for the proof that tobacco smoke is a cause of cancer had become overwhelming. Sir Derrick Dunlop, professor of therapeutics and clinical medicine at the University of Edinburgh, said in 1962, "To deny that cigarette smoking is an important factor in the etiology of lung cancer, peripheral vascular [blood vessel] disease, bronchitis, and probably coronary thrombosis is to carry skepticism to great lengths." Those who deny that cigarette smoking is the cause of lung cancer point to the many carcinogens in our polluted atmosphere. They say that as long as we are breathing these carcinogens, cigarette smoke cannot be blamed. But statistics show that pipe and cigar smokers have practically the same low incidence of lung cancer as do non-smokers.

Since there is no cure for lung cancer, the only weapon against it is avoidance. Admittedly, giving up the smoking of cigarettes is not easy, but there are many publicly available aids to doing so. Many a cigarette smoker has found it suddenly very easy to give up smoking when he is told he has lung cancer, but then it is too late.

Pulmonary Emphysema

Another respiratory disease that is commonly caused by smoking is pulmonary emphysema. This disease is characterized by shortness of breath and chronic cough. In the early stages breath is short only when the victim is walking or exerting himself in some other way. Later, he is short of breath even when sitting. Finally, his damaged lungs cannot transfer enough oxygen to his blood and death ensues.

Diet for Stomach Ulcers

Stomach ulcer, gastric ulcer, peptic ulcer, or simply ulcers, are another malady that is common in the United States. The cause of this disease is not clearly known, but for many years, ulcers were believed to be a result of continued tension in very active individuals, usually business executives. The standard treatment for ulcer patients was a diet containing bland foods and much milk. They drank milk about once an hour all day long. A recent study of ulcer patients, however, showed that those on a milk diet made no more progress than those who were not.

It was also found that hard-working business executives were far from the only ones suffering from ulcers. Housewives, store clerks, and even hoboes had about the same percentage of ulcers as the executives. A psychological cause was then suspected, and psychiatrists narrowed ulcer candidates down to the so-called oral dependent psychological type. Ulcers, then, were treated by psychotherapy. A fair number of cures were obtained by this treatment, so at least some stomach ulcers must have a psychological cause. But not all. When a case was not cured by psychotherapy, it was believed that the therapy had failed. No one suspected another cause.

In 1956, a medical journal contained an article on the treatment of 37 ulcer patients with concentrated cabbage juice. Ninety-two per cent of the patients were cured within three weeks; the other 8 per cent—those with the larger ulcers—were cured within five weeks.

Sometime later, a note appeared in the *Journal of the American Medical Association* in which the writer told of a number of ulcer patients who had been unsuccessfully treated with milk diet, antacids, antispasmodics, and tranquilizers. In desperation, they tried drinking cabbage juice and their symptoms cleared up.

Papaya juice also has been found to cure ulcers. It is not yet known what ulcer-curing substance both cabbage and papaya have in common, although some investigators have called it vitamin U (for "ulcer").

A recommended diet for ulcer sufferers includes a quart of cabbage juice a day, drunk between meals. Or, a 12-ounce can of papaya juice divided into four three-ounce doses, one at each meal and one at bedtime. Vitamin C should be taken in the form of sodium or calcium ascorbate instead of ascorbic acid, which may add to the acid condition of an ulcer patient's stomach. Also, a daily dose of vitamin B-complex should be taken. Smoking should be strictly avoided. So should spices and other strong seasonings which irritate the lining of the stomach.

Constipation: Simple Disease—Simple Cures

We have mentioned constipation in the section on body pollution by drugs. Here we look at causes and cures. Two very common causes of constipation are lack of water in the intestinal tract, and lack of bulk materials in the diet. Water passes through the walls of the small intestine and into the blood. The water is carried by the blood to the tissues that make up the organs of the body. When a person drinks a sufficient amount of water, the needs of the organs can be met and enough water left in the intestine to keep the undigestible part of the food and other body wastes in a moist and soft condition. This waste matter is easily moved through the intestines by their muscular contractions, and is eventually eliminated from the body by means of a bowel movement. If, however, a person drinks too little water, the needs of the organs are met by taking almost all the water from the undigested food and other wastes. This leaves a dry, hardened mass in the intestine, which the muscular movements cannot transport to the bottom of the lower intestine for elimination from the body. Constipation results. The cure is simple: eight glasses of water a day, two before breakfast.

Soft foods are those that contain a high proportion of water. Upon entering the intestine, most of the water is taken up by the blood and, after being used by the organs, is eliminated from the body by the kidneys. Since the soft food was mainly water, the undigested part left in the intestine is small in bulk. It therefore takes a long time—possibly a few days—for enough waste to collect in the lower intestine and provide the stimulus for elimination from the body. The result is constipation. The cure is foods higher in bulk materials that are undigestible. Examples are fresh fruits, eaten with the skins; vegetables, such as baked potatoes, also eaten with the skins, green beans, carrots, beets, peas, and broccoli; whole bran cereal, and whole wheat bread.

Remember that missing a bowel movement for a day or two is not cause for worry. If constipation persists after regulating your diet and you must have a laxative, try the natural ones: prunes and prune juice and raisins. If constipation continues, see a doctor. Don't dose yourself with laxative drugs from a drugstore.

Liver Disease

The liver is an extremely important organ. It forms bile, which is necessary for the proper digestion of fats; it converts the waste products of protein digestion into a form that can be eliminated by the kidneys; it completes the destruction of worn out red blood cells, produces an antianemic substance, and performs several other functions.

Liver cells depend on certain elements of the vitamin B-complex. Without these vitamin substances, the liver is not only unable to perform its functions, but the liver cells die from a type of malnutrition. The dead cells form tough, fibrous tissue and the liver shrinks in size. This situation is called cirrhosis, and may eventually lead to death.

Cirrhosis of the liver is a widespread health problem because it is connected with alcoholism, which afflicts at least eight million persons in the United States. Alcohol is a vitamin B antagonist which destroys the B-vitamin substances necessary for a healthy liver. Obviously, the best treatment for a person suffering liver damage from drinking too much alcohol is to stop drinking. This is not easy, and for some persons it may not be possible. Fortunately, the liver can repair damage to itself. If damage to a drinker's liver is not too great, he may be cured by large doses of vitamin B complex. Such doses should be taken only on the advice of a physician, and in most cases are given in hospitals.

If no liver damage exists, drinkers can insure against it. Dr. Paul de Kruif writes:

"If the nutritional treatment of advanced cirrhosis is so powerfully curative, why not use it to guard the liver while its cells are still normal? If we give our liver the right nutriments to work with, its cells will help to guard themselves. The nutritional supplements [the vitamin B-complex], added to a good diet, can be much like those used in the treatment of a sick liver—but less intensive and expensive. It takes far less to prevent liver failure than to relieve it. This preventive nutrition is a cheap price to pay for a strong liver—our best chance for top vitality."

Overweight and Undernourished

Next to dental caries, probably the most widespread body disorder is obesity. One authority estimates that at least one-fourth of the population of the United States over the age of three is overweight. There are more than 50 million persons who are over 10 per cent overweight; of these, more than five million are 20 per cent or more overweight.

Overweight men and women have a mortality rate 79 and 61 per cent, respectively, above normal. Overweight persons have more than $2\frac{1}{2}$ times as much diabetes as the rest of the population. Their death rates from cancer and heart disease are higher. Death from heart and blood vessel diseases among men 5 to 15 per cent overweight is 44 per cent higher than among men of normal weight. Among men 15 to 25 per cent overweight, the death rate from cardiovascular diseases is doubled. When we remember that these latter diseases kill more Americans than all other causes of death, the serious consequences of being overweight are frightening.

Although all the foregoing diseases may accompany or be caused by obesity, this condition is not a disease in itself. It is a symptom, an indication that something is wrong with the mechanism that balances the intake and utilization of food materials. In dealing with weight problems, the food intake is measured in terms of calories, which are units of heat energy.

In simplest terms, obesity is a condition in which more calories are taken into the body than are used up. The unused calories are stored in many places in the body as fat. Actually, the matter of obesity is not quite so simple. The endocrine glands play an important part in regulating the use of calories. For example, a person with an underactive thyroid gland may not eat more than he can utilize, yet the calories he does take in will be changed to fat at a cost to his general nutrition. He must learn to eat foods high in nutrients and low in calories.

Another complicating factor in the problem of obesity is the psychological one. A person's glands may be functioning normally and he may be able to afford a good diet—high in protein and low in fats and carbohydrates—yet he is overweight because he eats far more than he needs. Such a person probably is overeating for emotional reasons. That psychological factors are important in obesity is shown by the large number of overweight persons who find it impossible to summon up the will to cut down on the amount they eat.

Some obese people, desiring to reduce, simply go on a low-calorie diet and systematically lose weight. Such people are a minority. The nationwide existence of organizations that help people to reduce by means of a combination of diet and mild psychological devices proves that dieting is not a matter of simple will power for most people.

Doctors involved in managing overweight patients have found what has been termed "hidden hunger." Some patients who eat more than they need for their size, still complain of hunger. This hidden hunger has been found to be due to lack of vitamins and trace minerals in the diet. Persons whose diets have this lack are literally overfed, and according to nutritionist Moses Shedan, when persons suffering from hidden hunger are given nutritional supplements containing the missing vitamins and minerals, their hunger is dramatically lessened and they can then easily lower their calorie intake.

As we have learned, obesity may be caused by glandular imbalance or by psychological factors, as well as simply ingesting too many calories. The seriously overweight (fat) person who wishes to reduce should consult a physician to learn the cause of his rotundity. Simply deciding on a personal weight-losing method may be very harmful to fat people.

Persons with mild overweight problems will lose weight if they stick to the following program:

1) Restrict the amount of calories eaten to somewhere between 800 and 2000. Be careful not to cut down too drasti-

cally; the result of too great a cut may be malnutrition. If you feel weak, eat more and then cut down more slowly.

2) Keep carbohydrates—starches and sugars—and also saturated fats low in your diet.

3) Eat foods high in protein and low in saturated fats. Eat proteins in your breakfast. Eggs are not the only protein food that may be eaten at breakfast; fish and meat at breakfast are excellent foods with which the weight-reducer may start his day. Wheat germ is the best cereal for people on weight-loss diets. It contains only 125 calories per ounce; it has twice as much protein as an equal weight of fresh eggs, twice the iron of raisins, and more B vitamins and vitamin E than any other food; it also has unsaturated vegetable fats and 24 other vitamins, food elements, and minerals.

4) For insurance, take a daily dose of a multivitamin supplement that also contains the daily requirement of minerals.

5) Since dieting is difficult, you will find yourself tempted by appetite-suppressing preparations (which we discussed in the section on drugs) and tranquilizers. These should be shunned. If you feel you really need them, then you need a doctor's advice.

6) Strenuous exercise has no place in a reducing program. Such exercise may result in the loss of a few pounds immediately after it is over, but this loss is simply water that has been gotten rid of through perspiration. The exercise invariably generates a thirst which is satisfied by drinking liquids that return to the body the lost water and lost weight. Moderate exercise has a place in a reducing program, as it does in any health program, because it maintains good muscle tone and good circulation (which means good condition of the cardiovascular system), both of which help the body meet any stresses due to dieting.

The diseases we have surveyed make up far from a complete list of those that threaten the health of modern men and women. What is important is that almost all of these diseases can be cured by diet, including nutritional supplements. All diseases curable by diet can be *prevented* by diet, so several widespread diseases simply need not exist at all. A wide public knowledge of the principles of nutrition and their use plus a few other simple and natural measures could dramatically raise the level of health in the United States.

Emotional and
Mental Illness

Although tooth decay is the most prevalent disease in the United States and heart and blood vessel diseases kill more people than any others, our most serious medical problem is mental and emotional illness. More hospital beds are taken up by the mentally ill than by those with any other disease. The number of mental patients is increasing faster than those with all other illnesses combined. And mental patients are ill much longer than other sick persons.

The causes of mental, or emotional, illnesses are numerous and varied. Some mental illness is definitely caused by malfunctioning of the metabolism or by nutritional deficiencies and faults.

Thanks to the brilliant and dramatic discoveries of Sigmund Freud, the treatment of emotional problems and mental disease made a giant step forward. Out of Freud's work came the technique of psychoanalysis, in which the patient's personal history is uncovered in a large number of sessions in which he talks to the psychologically trained physician.

Freud, whose training was in medicine, taught that all patients with mental disorders must have a thorough physical examination before undergoing psychological treatment. He was aware that some symptoms which seem to be of mental origin actually are caused by physical factors such as brain tumors or by glandular imbalances. Too many of Freud's followers have forgotten this part of his teaching and ignore the physical basis of mental illness.

In the last few decades, evidence has piled up showing that the purely "talk therapy" of Freudian methods cannot cure a number of mental illnesses. It has been found that many of these illnesses are caused by inborn or acquired biochemical defects or deficiencies. A long-known example is oversecretion of the thyroid gland. A person suffering from this glandular malfunction is anxious and excitable to a degree that makes him mentally ill. Another example is schizophrenia, the most widespread of all serious mental illnesses. This disease is incurable by Freudian techniques. For about half a century, a small percentage of cures have been effected by electroshock therapy, and recently, psychiatrists have had considerable success in treating schizophrenia by means of massive doses of vitamins, and, as we shall see, by dietary therapy.

Blood Sugar and Mental Disorders

Dr. George Watson, a philosophy professor turned biochemist, has had some spectacular success in treating certain kinds of personality disorders by nutritional means. He has found that definite personality changes can take place when an individual's blood-sugar level is too low. This level is determined mainly by the individual's body chemistry. Two persons, having different body chemistries, who are given the same food in the same amounts, will have different levels of sugar in the blood after digesting the food.

Blood Sugar

Blood sugar gets its name from the fact that it is carried in solution by the blood to the cells of all the tissues of the body.

The importance of the blood-sugar level in mental health lies in the fact that the brain—which is functionally a very important part of the mind—derives its energy from blood sugar.

The energy is obtained as the sugar is oxidized, or burned, in the cells that make up the tissues of all organs of the body.

Another name for blood sugar is glucose. It is found pure in honey and grapes and a very few other foods. The body obtains most of its glucose by chemically transforming fruit sugar (fructose), milk sugar (lactose), carbohydrates (such as flour, cane sugar, starch, cereals), and certain proteins (such as meat, eggs, and fish).

Blood Sugar and Emotions

If blood sugar is not available, the cells of most organs can burn fat for energy. The brain cannot do this; it must have glucose. Thus the amount of sugar in the blood—the blood-sugar level—is very important to the brain. This organ uses as much as one-fourth of all the glucose in the blood, even though the brain makes up only about one-fiftieth of the total weight of the body.

If the blood-sugar level is too low and not enough glucose is available to the brain, marked personality changes take place. For example, normal emotional control is lost. This may first take the form of nervousness, depression, or unexplained weeping, and continue to violence, such as the desire to smash one's surroundings—or even to severe psychoses.

When an ordinary meal containing both carbohydrate and protein is eaten, the carbohydrate is fairly quickly transformed into blood sugar. The protein is digested more slowly, and that part which can be transformed into sugar is stored in the liver in the form of glycogen, or "liver sugar." After the glucose derived from carbohydrate is used up, the liver releases glycogen into the blood, transforming it to glucose. Protein alone cannot supply blood sugar, because the energy for the conversion of protein into glycogen must come from glucose which in turn comes from carbohydrate. Therefore, one must eat carbohydrate along with protein, if part of the protein is to be converted to glycogen.

To overcome the emotional symptoms resulting from low blood sugar, certain persons must learn how to eat a meal properly balanced between carbohydrates and proteins.

Doctors are familiar with the person who becomes nervous and depressed when on a reducing diet that is low in starch and sugar. This person is, of course, showing the symptoms of low blood sugar, but very few doctors are aware of the connection between the patient's diet and his emotional state.

The Oxidation of Blood Sugar

The use of glucose by the body's cells is not a simple process. Blood sugar is not burned directly; instead, the glucose is broken down into several substances, called intermediates. The important ones are acetyl coenzyme A, or acetate; and oxaloacetate, or o-acetate. Glucose mainly breaks down into o-acetate. Certain proteins and especially fats are sources of acetate; fats yield nearly twice as much acetate as protein!

The liver is the principal organ for transforming fat into acetate. But the liver can use very little of the acetate for providing energy. The excess acetate leaves the liver and is transported to other organs of the body which transform the acetate into energy.

The brain's ability to transform acetate into energy depends on the availability of substances that come from the oxidation of glucose, especially one substance called pyruvate. Thus, there is a dependent relationship between the amount of energy which the brain can obtain from acetate and the amount of glucose in the blood.

Enzymes and Energy Production

If the step-by-step breakdown of glucose in the brain is interfered with, the result will be impairment of mental processes. This is, of course, due to lack of glucose intermediates needed to oxidize acetate. At several points in the glucose-breakdown process, enzymes are needed. Lack of any of these enzymes interferes with the breakdown of glucose and can result in impaired mental functioning. For example, one such enzyme is the B-complex vitamin, niacin. In the section of this book headed "Diet and Skin," it was stated that one of the symptoms of pellagra is dementia, a mental illness, and that the cure for pellagra is a diet rich in the missing vitamin. By understanding the glucose-breakdown process and its significance in normal mental functioning, we can see why niacin deficiency can cause dementia. Lack of other vitamins and certain minerals also interferes with the processes involved in converting foods to energy and also may result in a variety of mental and emotional illnesses.

Slow Oxidizers and Fast Oxidizers

Some people are slow oxidizers and some are fast oxidizers. To understand how the metabolisms of slow and fast oxidizers differ, we have to know that there are actually two main cycles involved in the production of energy from food. One cycle, called glycolysis, is the one in which glucose in the blood is transformed into o-acetate and acetate. In the other cycle, o-acetate combines with acetate formed both from glucose and from fats and proteins. The second cycle is the citric acid cycle, which produces the energy in cells.

The fast oxidizer produces pyruvate and o-acetate faster than he produces acetate. He quickly oxidizes the acetate, and is left with unused pyruvate and o-acetate that cannot be converted into energy. The slow oxidizer's difficulty is the reverse: he does not produce enough pyruvate and o-acetate to oxidize the acetate he produces. In either case, there is an insufficient conversion of acetate into energy in the citric acid cycle. The fast oxidizer is not producing enough acetate; the slow oxidizer produces enough but cannot convert it to energy.

A Psychochemical Case

Dr. Watson details several cases of mental disorders which were cured by psychochemical, or nutritional, means. In summary, one case is the following.

A young woman had been diagnosed as having schizophrenia with periodic catatonia. She had been treated with both psychotherapy and electroshock. She had also received a number of drugs of the kind called "psychic energizers." In his first interview with her, Dr. Watson learned that before each catatonic attack, the patient "groped around" for a few days before she lost contact with reality. Dr. Watson assumed that the groping periods were ones in which, for some reason, there was a slowdown in the rate at which her metabolism was producing energy. Blood tests showed the patient to be a slow oxidizer. Dr. Watson gave her a diet and dietary supplements that increased her oxidation rate. The patient was then free of catatonic attacks for four months.

Thanks to the freedom from attacks, the patient went on a vacation in the High Sierras, doing much hiking and sloughing off her diet. As a result her oxidation rate fell and she started to enter a catatonic period. She was able to get back to Dr. Watson's clinic, where she was given intravenous injections of high-energy nutrients that pulled her out of the attack. However, before the injections were given, a blood sample was taken. It showed what Dr. Watson had surmised: she had a very low blood-sugar level.

After the patient was well for some months, she (at Dr. Watson's request) reversed her diet, eating for some days a diet that would normally be given to fast oxidizers—a diet that slows the oxidation rate. The result of the reversal was the onset of a catatonic attack. The circle was now closed: when the patient had low blood sugar, she experienced catatonic attacks; when her oxidation rate was increased, she was free of attacks; when she slowed her oxidation rate by means of diet, she brought on an attack. These facts left no doubt that the patient's mental illness was caused by metabolic malfunctioning coupled with the wrong diet for her type of metabolism. In other words, mental illness was caused by dietary deficiency and cured by proper diet.

Diagnosis and Diet

Dr. Watson has written a book about some of his work in psychochemistry. It is *Nutrition and Your Mind: The Psychochemical Response.* The book contains a section made up of 52 questions which may help the reader to establish his psychochemical type insofar as being a fast or slow oxidizer, or neither (normal). The basis for the questionnaire is that "unpleasant psychological reactions can directly and quickly result from wrong food choices." And "since one *can* choose a certain food, on the basis of taste alone, that will produce an adverse psychological reaction, one should always question a food choice which precedes any unusual emotional or mental response." The reader who answers the questions is told how to interpret them in deciding whether he is a fast or slow oxidizer, or neither. The results of the questionnaire point to a reader's *possible* psychochemical type: they do not insure it.

Dr. Watson points out that the only certain way to find an individual's psychochemical type is by means of a laboratory examination called a glucose tolerance test. In this test, the patient drinks a solution of 100 grams of glucose dissolved in 500 cubic centimeters of water flavored with lemon. Then, samples of his blood are taken every half-hour from three to six hours, and the level of glucose in each sample is measured. In patients who are fast oxidizers there will be a lowering of the amount of blood sugar in the first samples; in patients who are slow oxidizers, there will be a short-lived abnormal rise in the glucose level.

The diets prescribed for the fast and slow oxidizers are

based on what happens in the glycolysis and citric acid cycles of each type. Among the foods fast oxidizers are told to avoid or use very sparingly are candy, jams, jellies, ice cream, potatoes, bread, cereal, macaroni, spaghetti, spices, coffee, tea, and alcoholic beverages. Most of these foods are quickly converted to glucose which breaks down into more pyruvate and o-acetate than acetate. As a result, their energy is obtained and used quickly, leaving an energy deficit.

The slow oxidizer is told to shun pastries high in fat, Danish pastries, artichoke hearts, avocado, beans, peas, liver, kidney, brains, meat extracts, sardines, mussels, lard, butter, alcoholic beverages. Avoiding these foods prevents over-production of acetate which would not be converted into energy because the slow oxidizer cannot produce enough pyruvate and o-acetate to effect the energy conversion.

Nonfoods Psychochemical States

Dr. Watson and other researchers have found that personality changes and emotional disorders can be caused by other substances besides food. Pesticides, paint thinners, ammonia, mothballs, and other materials found around a house can trigger the undesirable mental conditions. This should not come as a surprise to anyone who remembers that if the step-by-step breakdown of glucose in the brain is interfered with, the result will be impairment of mental function. There are a large number of chemical substances that can cause this kind of interference. They need not be ingested in food, but can be breathed in or absorbed through the skin. Many of these substances are found in most households. Dr. Watson describes two cases of depression, one caused by naphthalene (mothballs and flakes) and the other by paint fumes.

One field that has yet to be explored is the psychochemical reactions caused by food additives. Research has revealed the physical damage done by additives, but practically no work has been undertaken to learn what influence these chemicals have on the mind.

Nutritional cures of emotional and mental illnesses offer great promise in the field of psychiatry, especially wherever the classical "talk therapy" has been consistently unsuccessful.

Alcoholism

One of the most serious forms of body pollution faced by modern man is alcoholism. In the United States and many countries of Eastern and Western Europe, alcoholism has reached epidemic proportions. In the United States, alcoholics have been estimated to number between eight and nine million. Tens of millions of man-hours of work are lost by alcoholics. They cause more than half of all the nearly 50,000 fatal automobile accidents each year. And the misery and tragedy in the lives of alcoholics and their families is beyond assessment.

The public's attitude toward the alcoholic has changed greatly in the last quarter of a century or so. Whereas an alcoholic was formerly considered to be a morally deficient individual of weak will, he is now widely understood to be a sick person. Authorities on alcoholism see this sickness as a complex problem with social, psychological, and nutritional aspects.

The social aspect includes the alcoholic in his relation to his family, friends, coworkers, and society in general, as when he causes an auto accident. The best response to an alcoholic's social problems is the association, Alcoholics Anonymous. This organization sets for its members the goal of total abstention from alcohol and strives to help them reach that goal by giving psychological support to them and their families through close association with former alcoholics.

The psychological aspect of alcoholism is considered by almost all authorities to be a part of the illness, yet a purely psychological approach to the cure of alcoholism has been so generally unsuccessful that most psychiatrists have thrown up their hands. This does not mean that psychotherapy has no place in the cure of alcoholism, but that it must be used in conjunction with other approaches.

In the last couple of decades, the possibility of treating alcoholism as a nutritional disease has gained importance. Dr. Roger J. Williams, a biochemist at the Clayton Foundation Biochemical Institute at the University of Texas, is a leading proponent of the nutritional attack on alcoholism. He applauds the social approach to alcoholism as a necessary part of a cure, and his book, *Alcoholism: The Nutritional Approach*, is dedicated to Alcoholics Anonymous. But Dr. Williams also gives weight to the psychological factors in the disease. His research has led him to believe that without the nutritional approach, which lessens the craving for alcohol, the alcoholic does not stand much chance of being cured by any other means.

What Is Alcoholism?

A simple definition of alcoholism is "the drinking of too much alcohol." But how much is "too much?" Some individuals can drink moderate amounts of alcohol habitually for decades without ill effects—that is, without harmful effects upon their work or family and social relationships. Others can drink immoderate amounts of alcohol—go on binges—every so often, also without permanent ill effects. Neither of these groups feels a constant craving for alcohol.

But there are others who do crave alcohol, who rely upon it like a god, and it is just this craving with its attendant damaging effects on an individual's body, his work, and human relationships which defines the "too much" of an alcoholic.

Alcoholism is a disease of individuals. Social groups do not suffer from alcoholism. Whole families, communities, or nations never become alcoholic. It is true that certain families seem to have more alcoholics than others, and that certain ethnic groups, such as the American Indians, show more than normal susceptibility to alcoholism. Yet, alcoholism strikes certain individuals in these groups and leaves others alone, even though all members may have equal exposure to alcohol.

One of the things that all alcoholics seem to have in common is the triggering action of a single drink. An individual who is not alcoholism-prone can take one or more drinks without craving more. When an alcoholic—even one who has abstained for a long time—takes a drink, he immediately craves another and another.

Another thing that seems to characterize an alcoholic is that the main interest in his life seems to be alcohol. Family, business, sex, friends, sports, intellectual pursuits, travel, politics, and every other activity that can enrich life have minimal value or none at all for an alcoholic. Simply urging an alcoholic to give up alcohol is bound to fail because it is asking him to give up the main desire in his life.

One of the ways to help an alcoholic is to try to get him (or her) interested in things other than alcohol. This kind of enrichment of life is one of the things that Alcoholics Anonymous does for its members and is one reason for the success this organization has had with alcoholics. Dr. Williams says, "In order to enrich people's lives, we need to know what their potentialities are and what enrichment they can take. You can enrich the life of a duck by giving it a pond in which to swim, but to enrich the life of a hen, keep her out of the wet and give her dirt to scratch in."

The Craving for Alcohol

Why does an alcoholic crave alcohol? It cannot be the taste. Although some people like alcohol, it is common to find alcoholics who detest its taste. This latter group drinks alcohol because, as most psychiatrists interpret it, alcohol enables them to escape from unpleasantness in their lives. However, there are persons with pleasant jobs and happy family lives who nevertheless become alcoholics. Another group of alcoholics whose members do not like the taste of alcohol are those who drink because they want to be members of an in-group which happens to be held together by "social drinking."

None of these reasons explains the constant craving for alcohol, the desire for one more drink to follow the last one, that is characteristic of alcoholics. Dr. Williams believes that alcohol is a physiological agent which causes the craving. The initial drink, acting physiologically on a "deranged cellular mechanism," produces the irresistible desire for more drinks. This desire is a kind of body-hunger like the dehydrated person's craving for water, or the intense need for salt of someone deprived of it.

A hangover, or "internal tremor," is definitely a physical— not a psychological—state. The true alcoholic will assuage his hangover with more alcohol, an action known as taking "hair from the dog that bit you." The alcoholic may be hungry when he wakes up to his hangover, yet he will not think of food, but of alcohol. Obviously, his normal body-hunger is being replaced by another, which is good evidence of deranged metabolism.

The Body's Control Mechanism

There are a number of automatic control mechanisms in our bodies. In the brain there is a temperature-control center which acts like a thermostat in maintaining a fairly constant temperature. When the body is too warm, the "thermostat" opens the pores which secrete water upon the surfaces of the body. This evaporating water cools the skin, including the millions of tiny blood vessels that form a network in the skin. The surface-cooled blood mixes with the rest of the blood and brings down the temperature of the whole body.

Also, the brain contains a respiratory center which controls breathing, activated by the amount of carbon dioxide in the blood. When there is a little more carbon dioxide in the blood than there should be, the blood is more acid than is normal. This triggers the respiratory center, which in turn activates the breathing muscles. The carbon dioxide is replaced by oxygen at an increased rate, and the blood returns to its normal alkaline-acid balance.

The automatic control mechanisms are similar in action to those that control the body-hungers for water, salt, and other nutrients. For example, the hypothalamus gland controls the weight of many individuals to a remarkable degree. The weight of most people does not vary more than ten pounds throughout most of their adult life. During this time, they eat thousands of pounds of food, yet it is digested and distributed in a constant way that keeps the body weight much the same throughout the whole period.

The control mechanisms are chemical in nature, as shown by the following example. Calcium and phosphorus metabolism is controlled by the parathyroid glands. The blood levels of these two elements are reciprocals; a high calcium level results in a low phosphorus level and vice versa. If the parathyroids of experimental animals are destroyed, the calcium level drops, and this induces a hunger for calcium and an aversion to phosphorus. A calcium-hungry animal will reject foods containing phosphorus.

Malfunctioning Control Mechanisms

The bodily control mechanisms by no means always work properly. This is commonly seen in those persons who gain too much weight on a diet that contains the normal amount of calories. An incorrectly functioning mechanism may be (1) anatomically malformed, (2) infected or poisoned by some agent being taken into the body, or (3) deficient biochemically in some nutritional factor it needs. A combination of these conditions may exist at the same time.

If a control mechanism is functioning poorly because of malformation, its owner can be given the chemical agent that is not being properly produced. For example, people with malfunctioning thyroid glands are given regular doses of thyroxin, the secretion of a normal thyroid. If infection or poisoning is the cause, the infection can be cleared up and the ingestion of poison eliminated. If the cause is a biochemical deficiency, it may be possible to supply the deficient factor, as in, for example, a vitamin B_1 deficiency.

In the last-mentioned of these three causes, malnutrition plays a very important part. Laboratory animals given diets poor in certain nutrients not only showed the effect of the deficiencies but went on to eat progressively poorer diets. This seemed to point to damage of the hunger control mechanism. For example, rats fed a nutritionally poor diet increased their intake of a sugar solution which was placed in their cages. The increased sugar consumption led the rats to choose a diet even more deficient in amino acids, minerals, and vitamins.

The foregoing seems to point to the fact that poor nutrition leads to further poor nutrition. It can also be shown that good nutrition leads to further good nutrition. Well-nourished animals, including human beings, have a "body wisdom" that leads to further good nutrition, while in malnourished animals, the body wisdom turns into body foolishness.

Biochemical Individuality

Each person is biochemically an individual. People may differ in (1) gross and microscopic anatomy, (2) blood composition, (3) enzyme levels, (4) endocrine gland activity, (5) excretion patterns, (6) response to chemicals, including drugs, and (7) nutritional needs. The variations may be as wide as 500 to 1000 per cent in normal individuals. For example, the gastric juice of one normal individual may have 400 times as much pepsin as that of another normal person. In abnormal persons, the variations are even wider.

Whenever a chemical substance (in food or drugs) has an effect on an individual, it is due to an interaction between the chemical and the body constituents of the individual. If the *same* chemical has a different effect on two people, it must be due to biochemical differences in the two persons. There are literally hundreds of documented examples to prove this statement.

Obviously biochemical individualism must be taken into account when explaining the physiological basis of alcoholism.

Genetotrophic Individuality

Equally as important as biochemical individuality is genetotrophic individuality. "Genetotrophic" means hereditary, or genetic, nutrition. A genetotrophic factor is one that involves an inherited bodily characteristic and its influence on nutrition. For example, a genetotrophic difficulty arises from the genetic possession of an unusually high nutritional need *plus* a failure to meet the need. If a rat on a standard diet develops a habit of drinking a large amount of alcohol (while his cage mates do not), and we can make the rat abstain by putting certain nutrients into its diet, we conclude that the desire is genetotrophic.

The connection between genetotrophic individuality and alcoholism is highly probable. Because of his genetotrophic background, an individual may have an abnormally high requirement for certain nutritional elements. Due to his biochemical individuality, the nutritional elements he needs will be peculiar to his genetotrophic requirements. When this person drinks alcohol in substantial amounts, he creates a nutritional deficiency in his body, because the alcohol serves as a substitute for necessary food elements such as minerals, vitamins, and amino acids. In certain cases, this deficiency causes cellular malnutrition in the tissues of the hypothalamus which damages the regulatory mechanism of this gland. Lack of regulation results in deranged body-hunger in which hunger for needed nutrients (foods) is distorted to a need for more alcohol. When this happens, no amount of reasonableness or will power can control the physiologically motivated urge to drink alcohol.

The Nutritional Treatment of Alcoholism

A person who has a genetotrophic difficulty that leads him to become an alcoholic can overcome his addiction to alcohol if his genetotrophically caused deficiencies are compensated for by a good basic diet and nutritional supplements. In other words, if a person has an inherited physiological difficulty that causes him to eat in a pattern that in turn causes him to develop a craving for alcohol, he can overcome his craving by proper diet. The whole group of symptoms and responses that make an alcoholic can be seen very well in experiments upon a population of rats.

First, the rats show much individuality in their response to alcohol when they are fed and treated alike in every way. The rats are fed a standard stock diet and are treated in a standard way. Some rats will not drink any alcohol although it is easily available to them for months. Others will drink a little every day for months, but never increase their intake. Others start with a little and slowly—in a period of several weeks—work up to consuming a large daily ration of alcohol. Others start with a small amount and work up to a large daily amount in a period of two weeks. Still others start at a high level and keep on consuming alcohol at this level. And some drink periodically, but heavily, for a day or two; then they abstain for a number of days before drinking again.

Second, the individuality in the rat's drinking pattern is genetically determined. The experimenters used a number of inbred, pure strains and found that each strain had its own drinking behavior pattern. This was accepted as proof that the urge to drink was determined by inheritance.

Third, the makeup of the rat's diets was a potent factor in determining the strength of their urge to drink alcohol. By making their diets deficient in a specific component vitamin, rats could be made to increase their daily consumption of alcohol five to thirty times. Then, by supplying their diets with the missing vitamin, the experimenters made the rats return to their original level of alcohol intake, or below. How well this dietary attack on alcoholism works depends on the individual animal.

Dr. Williams, whom we quoted at the beginning of this section, writes, "We cannot emphasize too strongly the fact that individual experimental animals having somewhat different ancestry, behave very differently with respect to alcohol consumption. Uniformly, they exhibit a physiological urge to drink when their diets are made deficient, but deficiency for one animal may be very different from deficiency for another. Some animals are very easily made deficient; others can tolerate what we regard as marginal diets very well by comparison."

All alcoholics who wish to attempt the nutritional approach must first "eat good nourishing foods, including high quality proteins [in meats, fish, poultry, eggs, and cheese] . . . vegetables, and fruits in accordance with the best nutritional knowledge. The diet ideally should also include one tablespoonful of corn oil . . . daily in salad dressing or other form." In addition to a good diet, the alcoholic should take a nutritional supplement of vitamins and minerals. Dr. Williams and his colleagues worked out the following formula for an effective supplement.

Thiamin (B_1)	3.30 mg
Riboflavin (B_2)	2.67 mg

Nicotinamide	20.00 mg
Calcium pantothenate (B_3)	20.00 mg
Pyridoxine (B_6)	3.30 mg
Biotin	0.05 mg
Folic acid	1.10 mg
p-Aminobenzoic acid	11.00 mg
Inositol	53.00 mg
Choline	53.00 mg
Vitamin B_{12}	5.00 μg
Vitamin A	6,667.00 units
Vitamin C	66.70 mg
alpha-Tocopherol	6.67 mg
Viosterol	333.00 units
Lipoic acid	0.10 mg

Another important item of the dietary supplement is glutamine, which alone had a consistent effect in decreasing alcohol consumption.

The recommended food supplement is sold under the names of Tycophan by the Eli Lilly Pharmaceutical Company, and as Nutricol by Vitamin-Quota, 1125 Crenshaw Blvd., Los Angeles, California 90019, or 880 Broadway at Nineteenth St., New York, N.Y. 10003. The dosage is three capsules per day with meals the first week, six per day the second week, and nine per day with meals the third week. After the cure has begun, the dosage can be lessened to the lowest number that still is effective.

The Psychological Factor

Although proper diet has effected cures of alcoholism, the percentage of cures is only fairly good. This can mean that much more knowledge is needed to make the dietary cures more effective, or that other factors are involved in alcoholism.

In Dr. Williams' laboratory, flashing lights and jingling cowbells working day and night were placed near the cages of rats. This annoyance caused teetotaler rats to begin drinking alcohol, even though they were on a diet that ordinarily kept them from having the urge to drink. Because these rats were actually "driven to drink," Dr. Williams stated that "stresses and annoyances can definitely increase the urge to drink alcohol."

Certain laboratories have found that stress-producing annoyances can increase the need for certain food elements, for example pantothenic acid. This fact points to the rats' need for alcohol as being physiologically produced. However, before the psychological factor can be ruled out we have to know at least two things. What causes the increased need for some dietary elements? Stress itself is psychological, so there *is* a psychological factor present. Second, would the consumption of alcohol end if the increased need for certain food elements were met by putting them into the rats' diets, while the stress-producing annoyances are still going on?

How Does the Cure Work?

In an article in the *Journal of the American Medical Association*, Drs. Trulson, Fleming, and Stare told of an experiment in which 32 alcoholics took part. Twenty-five were given vitamin medication and seven were given placebos [blanks]. "Of those taking vitamins, seven patients were abstinent, seven were controlled, two were improved, and nine exhibited no change, while of those taking the placebos, one was abstinent [a fact pointing to psychological motivation], and six exhibited no change." The authors say that not all the patients took the medicine faithfully, which lowers the possible effectiveness of the treatment. They concluded that "some persons are benefited by vitamin therapy." This is equivalent to passing a tough test, since Dr. Frederick J. Stare, one of the authors, has testified before Congressional committees in general opposition to the vitamin therapy advocated by nutritionists.

Although the percentage of cures is not very high, thousands of alcoholics have been cured by dietary therapy. The diet cure is very promising.

It is far from easy to bring most alcoholics to try the dietary (or any other) cure. According to Dr. Williams, the best promise for alcoholics is social and psychological help from Alcoholics Anonymous and psychological counseling to bring them to try the dietary cure.

Who Is Responsible?

We have described body polluting practices in the food, drug, cosmetics, fertilizer, and pesticide industries, and also among cattle, hog, and poultry raisers, and crop growers. These practices should leave little doubt that all Americans daily face a serious problem of eating a healthful diet while having to buy foods polluted with scores of chemical additives. Of not knowing which prescription or nonprescription drugs may do far more harm than good or may be simply worthless. Of risking healthiness of skin and hair when using cosmetics that can actually damage the parts of the body they are meant to enhance.

The worst aspect of this problem is that the consumer is almost helpless against those whose eagerness for profit presents him with the choice of body-polluting items in the supermarket or drug counter.

The Big Food Industry

Nearly 150 billion dollars' worth of food, detergents, and cosmetics are sold by food stores each year, according to an estimate by the Food and Drug Administration. This is about one-fifth of all the goods and services sold in the United States each year. The very rich food industry can and does afford a powerful public relations apparatus and lobby.

In 1960, Pulitzer Prize-winning ex-reporter William Longgood wrote *The Poisons in Your Food*, one of the first books to expose the dangers in food processing and in agriculture. Shortly after the book was published, checkers at most supermarkets were given pamphlets to put into one of the bags of every customer, along with the groceries and sales slips. Entitled "The Good in Your Food," the pamphlet assured supermarket shoppers that all was well as far as their health was concerned. The food in the brown paper sack was healthful and harmless. Additives were put into food to make it taste better, keep better, and look better, just as every shopper really wanted it to be.

The pamphlet came from the public relations staff of the Supermarket Institute. This group of executives, meeting in their 23rd annual convention, had felt that Longgood's book and other similar rumblings of discontent made public reassurance necessary. One supermarket executive said, "Our entire economy and way of life is based on faith. If faith in the wholesomeness of our food is undermined, it can have a serious effect on the health of our nation. It can seriously affect the public's confidence in government, agriculture, science, and education, as well as in manufacturers, processors, and distributors of food." To stem the possibility of this kind of national disaster, the pamphlet was written, printed in the tens of millions, and stuffed into brown paper bags.

The Food Association

There are a number of organizations encompassing most of the members of the food industry. These are nationwide groups with much money and a great amount of lobbying power. Among them are the American Meat Institute, National Livestock and Meat Board, American Dairy Association, National Dairy Council, Wheat Foods Association, Wheat Flour Institute, Cereal Institute, and Sugar Research Foundation, Inc. The words "institute," "board," "council," and "foundation" give these public relations and lobbying organizations an odor of respectability that screens their true purposes.

The Sugar-Coated Bamboozle

Almost all of these organizations carry on some research into the uses of the particular kinds of food each represents. They also subsidize research in universities and research institutes. It is hard to say how much this research benefits any part of the population besides its sponsors, but one thing certain is that research which turns up findings unfavorable to sponsors rarely sees the light of publication.

The Sugar Research Foundation provides an example. This trade organization was founded in 1937 by 77 sugar producers and refiners of cane and beet sugar in the United States and other countries. Since its foundings, its membership has more than doubled. Its publication, *Sugar Molecule*, explained one of its research purposes thus: "The purpose of our dental caries research is to find out how tooth decay may be controlled effectively without restriction of sugar intake." In the Institute's search for an answer, it supported work by James H. Shaw and associates, biochemists, for more than ten years. At the Harvard School of Dental Medicine, the researchers explored the effects of sugar on the teeth of laboratory animals. One population of rats was fed a sugar-rich diet, while a control group was put on a sugar-free regimen. The results were what one might expect—the control group showed almost no cavities (Look, Mom, no cavities!), but the rats on the sugar diet suffered many. From these results, Dr. Shaw reported that "we should cut down on our sugar consumption, particularly candy. We should be careful about sugars that remain in the mouth because of their physical properties."

This report ended the research project because it prompted the Sugar Research Foundation's financial withdrawal. The results of the experiments were published in the esoteric *Journal of the American Medical Association*, but never appeared where the public would be likely to see them.

The Sugar Research Institute spends large amounts of money on advertising the idea that sugar gives one quick energy, a fact that is entirely false, according to the hitherto mentioned work of Drs. Yudkin and Watson. The Institute also gives aid to soft drink bottlers who are trying to neutralize the efforts of an increasing number of dentists who warn their patients that beverages containing sugar are not good for the teeth. Furthermore, the S.R.I. urges canners to use 60 per cent more sugar "to gain maximum consumer acceptance," a successful campaign that has resulted in the virtual impossibility to get—except in health food stores—fruits canned in their own juices, rather than the thick syrups used by the large canners.

The Nutrition Foundation, Inc.

In 1941, the leaders of the food industry formed the Nutrition Foundation, Inc. Companies that were director-members included American Can, American Sugar Refining, Beechnut, California Packing, Campbell Soup, Coca-Cola, Container Corporation, Continental Can, Corn Products Refining, General Foods, General Mills, H. J. Heinz, Libby, McNeill, & Libby, National Biscuit, National Dairy Products, Owen-Illinois Glass, Pillsbury Flour Mills, Quaker Oats, Safeway, Standard Brands, Swift, and United Fruit.

Sustaining members included Abbott's Dairies, American Home Foods, American Lecithin, Bowman Dairy, Continental Foods, Crosse & Blackwell, Curtiss Candy, R. B. Davis, William Davis, Drackett, Flako, Gerber, Golden State, Hansen Laboratories, Knox Gelatine, McCormick, Minnesota Valley Canning, National Sugar Refining, Nut & Chocolate, E. Prichard, Red Star Yeast, Stouffer, Weston, and Zinsmaster. Financial contributions came from American Maize Products,

A&P, Hawaiian Pineapple, Eli Lilly, Merck, Penick and Ford, and A. E. Staley.

We have risked boring you with this long list of companies in order to give you an idea of what the financial resources of the Nutrition Foundation, Inc. are, and what lobbying power they can wield. The Foundation sponsors' research into many aspects of nutrition through grants to medical and dental schools and other university departments. It cannot be denied that some valuable findings have come out of this research. However, control over the direction and dissemination of results is maintained by the Foundation. Since the findings of the research do not ever embarrass the Foundation members in their manufacturing and marketing activities, there is much reason to suspect that many research reports never see the light of publication.

Science in the Service of Pollution

One of the largest recipients of money from the Nutrition Foundation is the Department of Nutrition at Harvard University, headed by Dr. Frederick J. Stare. Dr. Stare has impressive academic qualifications and his administrative ability is obvious. Yet, he is the author of the following statements:

"Sugar is a quick energy food. . . . Even people on a severe reduction diet can afford to put a teaspoonful of sugar in their tea or coffee three or four times a day."

"The nutritive qualities of canned evaporated milk are every bit as good as those of fresh pasteurized milk." (In April 1964, Dr. Stare was elected a member of the board of directors of the Continental Can Company.)

An after-school snack for teenagers recommended by Dr. Stare is "iced tea, lemon- or limeade, or Coke."

These statements should lead one to wonder whether Dr. Stare has the time to do much reading in his own field, since there is a considerable amount of sound research that contradicts his pronouncements.

Dr. Stare is not the only scientist who serves a dual role as a member of the food industry and as a researcher in the academic world. Once a scientist enters such a relationship, he becomes something less than a scientist—an impartial, objective searcher for truth. He usually ends up as a mouthpiece for the food industry.

One of the results of industry-sponsored research is the existence of a number of apologists for food industry processing practices. Dual-role scientists are continually testifying at congressional hearings and are almost invariably found pooh-poohing the possible dangers of food additives and other adulterants, as well as nutrition-decreasing processing practices.

That the Nutrition Foundation is not in existence primarily to encourage research in nutrition is easily seen in its public relations activities, which expend more than a million dollars a year. It sends "informational" stories on nutrition to newspapers. Also, editorial material is sent to trade journals and consumer magazines which have an estimated total readership of more than 50 million.

The project, Dial-a-Dietician, which was begun in Detroit in the late fifties, was launched with money from the Nutrition Foundation. Any consumer who dials an advertised phone number is given nutritional information—information that assures him the food available at the usual markets is wholesome, nutritional, and safe.

When William Longgood's *The Poisons in Your Food* was published, Dr. William J. Darby, a nutritionist, led an attack on the book. He was joined by Dr. Charles Glen King. Dr. Darby was the recipient of grants from the Nutrition Foundation, and Dr. King was planner and first director of the Foundation, and later its president. Dr. King had also led the attack on Rachel Carson's *Silent Spring*.

A continual flow of propaganda, in the guise of helpful nutritional information, goes to newspapers, magazines, and trade journals. It is impossible for the nutritionally untrained reader to sift truth from falsehood in this flood of information, and even the trained reader must do much searching to straighten out the material that comes from the Nutrition Foundation's public relations mill.

The U.S. Government and the Food Industry

In 1958, Congress passed the Food Additives Amendment, Public Law 85-929. This law was the result of lengthy hearings conducted by Representative James J. Delaney. In 1949, when Rep. Delaney first announced these hearings, the Food and Drug Law Institute (FDLI) was formed. It had as sponsors just about all the members of the food industry who were involved in the Nutrition Foundation.

The FDLI has on its roster of officials "public members" who came from government, especially those agencies charged with administering and enforcing the food laws. The officers of FDLI come from the food industries, and among them are "public trustees" like Dr. Darby, Dr. King, and other officers of the Nutrition Foundation.

The FDLI sponsors and pays for courses on food, cosmetics, and drug laws given in law schools because it wishes "to give sound advice to industry and government," so that "existing laws [can] be understood and observed and that amendments [can] be carefully considered and adopted only when sound and in the public interest."

Those invited to attend these instructions include industry and government lawyers. This means, in the words of consumer advocate Beatrice Trum Hunter, that "the FDLI plays an important role in the drafting and interpreting of all legislation dealing with consumer protection in the areas of food, drugs, and cosmetics."

The FDLI also sponsors lectures, seminars, and conferences on food and drug laws. It publishes a journal and legal research texts, and maintains liaison with government agencies, universities, and domestic and international bar associations. Its information sources, legal skills, and technical knowledge are used at public hearings on food and drug laws. In short, FDLI is a wealthy, technically expert, widely connected lobby for the food and drug industry.

Whose Hats Are They Wearing?

As we learned in the section on MER/29 and Kevadon-Thalidomide, there is a very relaxed, fraternal relationship between some of the government regulatory agencies and the industries that the agencies are supposed to regulate. Officials are continually leaving government service to become highly paid executives in the industries they were formerly charged with regulating. Their associates who are zealous in guarding the public interest by strictly interpreting government regulations are not likely to end up with lucrative offers from industry.

Also, people from industry join government regulatory agencies for a time and then return to industry. The enthusiasm of such officials for guarding public interest at the possible expense of their former and future employers is not likely to be great.

There are many joint government-industry-public commissions and committees that act in an advisory capacity to government regulatory agencies or congressional committees. In these joint groups it is presumed that the industry members and government members will not act in any way that will hurt the interests of their respective agencies. This leaves only the public members for the position of the public's advocates. However, when the public members are closely scrutinized, a surprising number turn up as members of the foundations, institutes, and boards which are supported by industries.

Scientists for Sale

In the hearings before the House Select Committee to Investigate the Use of Chemicals in Food and Cosmetics (82nd Congress, 2nd session), Leonard Wickenden, an industrial chemist, testified:

"I have upon my desk an advertisement published by the National Fertilizer Association. I think it is fair to call it a typical advertisement. From beginning to end it is extremely biased. Its byline reveals that it was written by a distinguished professor on the staff of one of our more important agricultural colleges. If some of the professors in our agricultural colleges are employees of the National Fertilizer Association, or of any of its members, can we be quite confident that their teaching is entirely unbiased? If some of the members of the staffs of our state experiment stations are receiving compensation in any form from the same source, can we be fully satisfied that all their research work is wholly in the interest of the farmers and to no slightest degree in the interests of the manufacturers of poison sprays, or other materials or equipment used in agriculture?"

The point that Wickenden raises is not only valid when judging the work of academics in their own fields, but also concerns government because the faculty members of colleges and universities are almost always to be found on governmental regulatory agencies' advisory boards. Also, they are among the most frequently called expert witnesses at congressional hearings. In the sciences almost all who teach or do research in universities are in some way connected with the National Academy of Sciences' National Research Council. This quasi-governmental agency is frequently called upon to perform tasks for the national government, such as appointing committees to review problems of public interest. For example, in 1966 the Department of Agriculture asked the NAS-NRC to appoint a Committee on Persistent Pesticides to investigate this problem, especially as it applied to DDT. More than 80 witnesses testified before this committee, nineteen of whom were ecologically oriented. Another nineteen were from the industries that made the hearings necessary in the first place. Three witnesses were from the food industry, fourteen from the public health field, and twenty-eight from agriculture (who planned agriculture's commitment to DDT!).

After hearing these witnesses, the committee did not recommend any kind of ban on DDT, but recommended further study of the problem.

There is a Committee on Pest Control and Wildlife Relationships within the NAS-NRC. It includes 43 "supporting agencies," of which 19 are chemical corporations and four are trade organizations. In 1962, this committee issued two reports. Upon reading them, Dr. Frank Egler, an ecologist, wrote:

"The problem of industries' influence on scientists who are on their payrolls as consultants, through research grants and otherwise, is a prickly one. It has been brought up in connection with these reports. My surprise is not that such influence exists, but that other scientists are so naive and unsophisticated as to refuse to believe it. The reader should at least know of such connections in appraising the final conclusions. In short, these two [reports] cannot be judged as scientific contributions. They are written in the style of a trained public relations official of industry, out to placate some segments of the public that were causing trouble. With different title and cover pages, they would serve admirably for publication and distribution by a manufacturers' trade associations. Indeed, they are being much quoted in such places." ("Pesticides and the National Academy of Scientists," *Atlantic Naturalist*, Oct.-Dec., 1962.)

Unnecessary Protection

In 1960, an article by Dr. E. V. Askey, a past president of

the American Medical Association (AMA), appeared in the *Journal of the American Medical Association.* The article was titled, "Americans Wasting Millions on Vitamins." Dr. Askey said, "Americans have to go out of their way nutritionally speaking, to avoid being well-nourished." He went on to say that most citizens get all the vitamins they need in their daily diets, and that supplementing their daily food intakes with vitamins is a waste of money. Dr. Askey was strangely silent or ignorant about concurrent nationwide surveys that showed large percentages of Americans of all ages and all economic levels to be eating diets deficient in one or more nutrients, according to the Recommended Daily Allowances published by the NAS-NRC's Food and Nutrition Board. Of course, the food industry grabbed Dr. Askey's statement and gave it the widest publicity.

Dr. Askey's statement was only one event in a continuing campaign against the use of vitamin (and mineral) supplements. In 1962, the late George P. Larrick, then the FDA Commissioner, proposed regulations that would prohibit the sale or purchase of vitamins except by a doctor's prescription or in very small amounts. The FDA did not contend that the vitamins were harmful, which would have been the only justification for the proposed regulations. Instead, they repeated Dr. Askey's general contention that the average American diet provides all the vitamins an individual needs and therefore purchase of supplementary vitamins is a waste of money. What Commissioner Larrick wanted to do was to force Americans to spend (or not spend) their money in ways he saw fit. He did not cite any statute that gave his agency this power.

He also did not explain how anyone would save money by first paying for a doctor's prescription and then buying the vitamins at prescription drug prices, which are about 30 times as much as when bought over the counter.

The FDA went to the news media and gave them its views on vitamins and nutritional supplements, hoping to use the news media to win its case before any hearing on the proposed regulations were held. This move did not work because the news media did not have enough influence with the public. Also, consumer groups, such as the National Health Federation, were keeping the public aware of the FDA's moves. As a result, Commissioner Larrick drew back and temporarily shelved his proposal.

The regulations to "protect" the consumer against buying any vitamins he might need remained on the shelf until Dr. James Goddard succeeded Larrick. Commissioner Goddard revised the regulations, tightening them by giving the FDA even more control over the sale and purchase of vitamins and nutritional supplements. Every label that was to go on vitamins and dietary supplements was to bear the following:

"Vitamins and minerals are supplied in abundant amounts by commonly available foods. Except for persons with special medical needs, there is no scientific basis for recommending routine use of dietary supplements." Originally, there had been more to the label: "The Food and Nutrition Board of the National Research Council recommends that dietary needs be satisfied by foods." This statement was deleted because the Food and Nutrition Board insisted that *it had never made such a statement* and that use of its name was unauthorized. Dr. LeRoy Voris, Secretary of the National Research Council, said that the Food and Nutrition Board had never reviewed nor approved the assertion attributed to it by the FDA; what is more, there never was, as far as he knew, any discussion of that matter between the FDA and the Board.

Other members of the Food and Nutrition Board also complained. For example, Dr. W. M. Sebrell, Jr., wrote, "This statement is objectionable and misleading, and uses the authority of the Food and Nutrition Board . . . to support a statement which, taken out of context, creates a false impression.

"The generalization that vitamins and minerals are supplied

in abundant amounts in the food we eat has no relevance as applied to a particular individual." In other words, how does the FDA know whether *you* get enough vitamins and minerals in what *you* eat?

Dr. Sebrell took exception to the part of the FDA-proposed label that said "special medical needs." He said that "there must be many thousands of people in this country on restricted diets for the purpose of losing weight who do not have any serious medical need, but who should take vitamins because of the limitations of their foods intake." And "there are certainly many thousands of people on special diets of other kinds for various reasons, medical and non-medical, for whom there would be a scientific basis for dietary supplementation."

Concerning the FDA's claim that Americans were getting all the vitamins needed in their daily diet, Dr. Thomas H. Jukes, lecturer in nutrition at the University of California, said, "I do not think any professor of nutrition would give a passing grade to a student who made such a statement."

Another nutritionist, Dr. Steve Weider of Kissimmee, Florida, said that the FDA's decision to ban nonprescription vitamins was "an abominable absurdity, since most Americans eat processed foods which have lost their vitamins and minerals in the processing."

Dr. Ray Morey of Marietta, Ohio, Henry Burke Health Institute reminded the FDA that such a decision to restrict vitamins on the commercial market would affect food processors, also. Most of them "enrich" their foods adding some of the vitamins that are lost in processing. The Campbell Soup Company and the H. J. Heinz Company wanted to continue over-fortifying their fruit juices with vitamin C to make up for the amount lost in storage.

After two years of behind-the-scenes foot-dragging, the FDA opened hearings on the proposed regulation. Most of the witnesses were persons hand-picked by the government.

The FDA's attorneys expressed an aversion to having all

sides of the question aired. In the proceedings, at least one focus of the FDA's bias against the health food industry emerged. Sidney Weissenberg, assistant associate Commissioner for Compliance, ranted against "so-called health food stores," "food faddists," and "quacks." Mr. Weissenberg spent 52 days on the witness stand—longer than any other witness. When he was told to desist from using the phrase "so-called health food stores," he ignored the examiner's order.

It turned out that he was a one-man board of censorship of what could and could not be printed on vitamin containers. "It is Mr. Weissenberg who first makes that determination," a government attorney testified. "FDA relies on him to do this . . . every day with no guidelines . . . that is what we bring our cases on." The FDA attorneys showed Weissenberg a number of vitamin labels which had been handpicked to make the government's point, but it turned out that Weissenberg could not tell which were in current use.

One of the more vicious of the FDA's maneuvers at the hearing was to try to make it impossible for the opposition to get transcripts of the proceedings. The FDA entered into a contract with the Columbia Reporting Company, of Washington, D.C., to buy the transcript at nine cents a page, but allowing the company to charge consumer groups and industry representatives 75 cents a page, a price most could not even come near paying.

Dr. Frederick J. Stare turned up in opposition to the FDA. He wrote the Examiner, "Strange as it may seem, we have little factual information on the present nutritional status of representative groups of people in our country." And, using the testimony of Surgeon General Dr. William Stewart, when he appeared before a Senate investigating committee in 1967: "We do not know the extent of malnutrition anywhere in the United States—I cannot say what the extent is, because we just don't know," Dr. Stare continued, "With such a clear statement from the head of our Public Health Service, a statement with which most physicians knowledgeable in nutrition would agree, I don't see how anyone at this time can intelligently recommend new regulations on special diet foods, vitamin and mineral fortified foods and supplements." Dr. Stare went on to urge that the hearings be recessed until more knowledge on the nation's nutritional status could be obtained. The hearings continued.

In January 1970, the new FDA Commissioner Charles C. Edwards ordered the hearings ended in time to have a report ready by June 1. The Examiner announced that all testimony of opponents of the regulation had to be in by March 16. This meant that the FDA had 16 months in which to present its testimony, but the opponents (104 of them) would have to rush through their case in three months.

The foregoing account of the FDA's attempt to outlaw the over-the-counter sale of vitamins and minerals as food supplements has been described in some detail (regretfully leaving out a number of underhanded and even illegal actions on the part of the FDA) because it is typical of the FDA's attitudes and actions in its handling of health-related matters that stem from its bureaucratic ideology. Most important, it shows the FDA's dictatorial methods used against those who disagree with that ideology.

When the long and expensive hearing came to an end in early 1971, the FDA had not won the labeling victory it had sought; the results were inconclusive. But the FDA does not give up easily. On December 12, 1972, the FDA proposed restrictions on the potency of vitamins. The proposal was to limit vitamin A to 10,000 international units and vitamin D to 400 units per capsule or other unit dosage. The FDA said the restrictions would apply to "vitamin products marketed as foods for special dietary purposes and as over-the-counter drugs."

The Associated Press dispatch said, "Americans have been taking vitamin supplements for decades, but concern has been heightened by the new health-food craze."

The FDA announcement said that persons interested in the proposed restrictions have 60 days to comment on them. Also, these restrictions will be followed "in the near future" by broad regulations covering most other vitamins, minerals, and other food supplements.

The AP dispatch ended, "The FDA is said to be considering rules setting minimum and maximum amounts of nutrients in multivitamins and mineral products, prohibiting health claims, and requiring expiration dates on labels." The AP writer did not know that this really was not news.

Perhaps one more example should be given. The account comes from the preface written by Dr. George W. Crane to the book, *The Dictocrats' Attack on Health Foods and Vitamins*, by Omar V. Garrison. At a famous FDA trial, a Justice Department attorney, who was not assigned to the case, asked one of the defendants, "Doctor, do you know why *you* were indicted? Especially since the government knew you were merely a neutral professor who had offered free advice as you would to any other scientist who might seek out your counsel. So why do you think you were indicted?"

"I've often wondered," the good doctor replied, "*why* did the government include me in the indictment?"

"Well, that's standard procedure," replied the Washington attorney. "The government knew that sooner or later you would be called into court as an expert witness for the defense, since you are the world's foremost physiologist and researcher.

"So the government indicted you to discredit any testimony you might make. It's part of our strategy to reduce the credibility of opposing witnesses!

"The average American thinks 'indictment' is synonymous with 'being guilty.' So our Department of Justice spreads its indictments over all possible witnesses for the defense!"

This horror tale, aside from being an account of something that one would expect in a totalitarian government, and not in the United States, should cause one to ask just what tactics like that on the part of the FDA have to do with this agency's purpose, which is to protect the American citizen from unsafe drugs, dangerous additives and pesticide-engendered poisons in his food.

The News and Advertising Media

Since the time of Thomas Jefferson, the citizens of this country have been told countless times that a free and impartial press is one of the main bastions of our liberty. Fortunately for us, and despite its many shortcomings, our press is free and doing a good—though far from perfect—job. Those who know something about the news media (of which, the press is, today, but one segment), are aware that the good things that emanate from the media are the work of a minority of the reporters and editors who are gathering, interpreting, and disseminating news. The rest follow the herd and do as little work as possible, and they are the main targets of news services that give information on events, policies, and persons in and out of government. What is important to us here is that reporters who rely on news services necessarily reflect the viewpoint of news services. And news services get much of their information from printed handouts.

The FDA, in its vendetta against health food makers, distributors, stores, and literature, grinds out scores of handouts castigating the whole health food enterprise as a huge crackpot venture. Thus, in the autumn of 1972, when, as we saw above, the FDA opened another round in the Battle of the Vitamins, the Associated Press dispatch spoke about the "health food craze." It was easier for the Associated Press reporter to accept the stereotyped description of the health food movement than to find out something about it himself. This one instance is typical. The majority of the news media docilely goes along with the opinions of the health food movement that are held by the government agencies and the industry lobbies.

Omar Garrison tells of a raid made by FDA agents and state food inspectors upon a small Detroit department store. The raiders seized a supply of safflower oil capsules, claiming that they were being used to promote the sale of a book, *Calories Don't Count*, from which the FDA wanted to "protect" the consumer. The *Detroit Free Press* ran a front-page story of the raid and accompanied the article with a four column photograph captioned, "Store employees look on as government agents seize 'reducing capsules.'" The newspaper story failed to give a reasonably equal account of the small department store's side of the raid.

In 1965, the then FDA Commissioner James Goddard disclosed that his agency was distributing through a trade-union news agency "news articles" [handouts] giving the FDA's viewpoint on drugs and cosmetics. The stories were written by a free-lance writer working under contract to the FDA, not by any member of the working press. As printed in newspapers, the articles gave no clue that they were prepared for a government agency under its direction, and were not news stories at all.

The *Wall Street Journal* commented on this sneaky practice, "To be sure, it is not likely anybody has been done any serious harm by FDA's bashfulness about being identified as the source of this 'news' it is giving away free—the question is whether it is proper for any governmental agency to feed this propaganda in disguise to a segment of the press gullible enough to accept it."

In 1967, Princeton University Press published *The Medical Messiahs: A Social History of Health Quackery in Twentieth Century America*, by James Harvey Young. In the preface, Mr. Young stated that his research and writing had been supported over a span of years by a Public Health Service Research Grant. The grant also provided Mr. Young with a research assistant.

This practice is a double fraud. Public funds were being

used to pay a writer to produce a book under the auspices of the government. The book, which reflects the viewpoint of its governmental sponsor, is then published under the imprint of a commercial publishing house. Thus, the first fraud has been perpetrated. The taxpayer who buys the book has paid for its production with his tax dollars, then he pays for it a second time when he buys it. Thus, a second fraud.

Using the FDA Properly

The Food and Drug Administration is not a very large government agency as government agencies go, yet it has thousands of employees throughout the country. Most are in Washington, D.C., but a considerable number are spread out in many cities to make it convenient for the FDA to carry on its work of inspecting food, drug, and cosmetic producers.

The need for the FDA is obvious. With thousands of food additives available to food processors and more thousands of drugs and cosmetics on the market, and with scores more of these items continually being introduced, an impartial agency is needed to protect the public from poisonous, useless, and worthless foods, drugs, and cosmetics. The Food and Drug Administration is the governmental agency created by Congress to impartially and fairly carry out this work of protection.

The job the FDA has been given is vast. There are more than 2,500,000 interstate shipments of fruits and vegetables each year in the United States. The FDA is able to inspect only 1 per cent of this food. The reason is lack of inspectors.

The FDA has to inspect about 90,000 food processing establishments for cleanliness and for the ingredients that go into the processed food. The FDA has the manpower to inspect only one-fourth of the processors. That there is a need for such inspection is emphasized by the 80,000,000 pounds of food seized each year for filth, decomposition, and unsanitation of the premises.

Each year, nearly 400,000 shipments of foodstuffs, cosmetics, and drugs enter the United States from other countries, some lacking almost any health and sanitary laws.

A recent FDA commissioner revealed that his agency receives, on an average working day, four applications for approval of drugs; eight proposals for the testing of new drugs; and 13 requests for modification of drugs previously approved. The processing of a single application may take almost 200 work days, involve 29 members of the FDA, six outside consultants, and 19 other outside contacts; also conferences, laboratory tests, and field trips. The record of this typical application may run to 4,000 pages.

Of the 14,000 drug establishments that the FDA must inspect, it can get around to only half each year. The Commissioner said, "This is far from adequate coverage of an industry whose output is so closely associated with the health and well-being of every citizen." One result this situation causes is a great number of drug-induced deaths and permanent injuries due to drugs which are suffered by patients each year. We have seen some of them in the story of MER/29.

Every American citizen owes the Food and Drug Administration a debt, because most of its overworked staff do an honest and valuable job of protection. The competence and dedication of Dr. Frances Kelsey, who saved American women from the nightmare of Thalidomide-deformed children, are not exceptional in the FDA.

On the other hand, we have seen in this book how some employees are blindly prejudiced against the health food industry and command a large staff of agents and inspectors in a Gestapo-like war of extermination on the objects of their prejudice. We have seen, in the case of the vitamin hearings, how the FDA's legal staff can engage in patently dishonest tactics that deny some of the basic freedoms that are the right of every American citizen. How readily and eagerly the FDA will take destructive confiscatory action against a small health food store for allegedly mislabeling a few bottles of honey, but then do nothing about confiscating several hundred thousand bottles of wine mislabeled by a large vintner. It is these things— very, very serious things—that give a useful and desperately needed agency a bad reputation.

Since the Food and Drug Administration has so important a part to play in the life of every citizen, all citizens should be concerned with making the FDA work properly. Unfortunately, most citizens are ignorant of the problem and many who have any knowledge of it are indifferent. The burden of taking action then falls upon a few thinking, concerned citizens. That the probability of reforming the FDA is not as remote as it may seem, and how it might be done can be seen as we read in the next section about what has already been done.

Taking Action

If what you have read so far upsets you, you are not alone. Millions of other American consumers are outraged by the pollution of our soil by pesticides and chemical fertilizers. They are frightened by the additives in the foods they and their children are forced to eat. Almost weekly, there are news reports of poisonings by food additives, or laboratory reports that another additive has been found to cause cancer. Consumers are angered by the bureaucratic highhandedness of the administrative and legal department of the Food and Drug Administration and other government agencies. As short a time as five years ago, the unhappy consumer could do little more than look on in frustration at the body-polluting situations that seemed to surround him. Today, he no longer needs to feel frustrated; there are constructive channels into which he can turn his anger and do something to fight body pollution.

Consumerism

The anti-pollution movement is a broad one. It includes action against not only those who pollute our bodies through foods but also through air filled with gaseous industrial wastes and automobile emissions, as well as lakes and streams fouled by solid and liquid industrial wastes and sewerage. This is part of a broad ecological movement.

The anti-pollution movement is allied with those who are tired of being cheated by large corporations that sell shoddy and unsafe merchandise, from children's toys to automobiles. This part of the movement is consumerism, and it includes action against the manufacturers of harmful and useless foods, drugs, and cosmetics.

The consumer movement has been a long time growing. It would be difficult to say just when this movement began. If a single event were to be picked as a beginning, it might be the publication in 1928 of a book titled *100,000,000 Guinea Pigs*, by Kallet and Schlink. This book made the reader aware of the great differences in the quality of the goods he was buying and how the manufacturers treated the average consumer as if he were a guinea pig on which to try out the sale of ill-made, harmful, or useless goods. From this book sprang a consumer goods testing organization, Consumers' Research, Inc., which published a monthly bulletin telling subscribers the results of the product tests. This enabled the consumer to exert a little influence by purchasing only the products that were reported to be healthful or well-made. In 1936, Consumers' Research split and a new testing organization, Consumers Union of the U.S., Inc., was founded. Today, the younger organization has become the larger, but both testing organizations are functioning and satisfying the consumer's desire for impartial product advice.

At first, the testing organizations were met with skepticism by many consumers, who believed that the testers were paid by manufacturers to certify products as being good buys, and the business community showed hostility to the product testers. But, these attitudes have largely been dispelled by the procedures used by the two research organizations: unannounced purchases of samples in the open market; refusal of permission to any company to use test results in its advertising; scientifically impartial testing procedures; allowing the members (subscribers) to elect the board of directors and to propose the products and services to be tested. Also, Consumers Union gives voice to its members' complaints against deceptive advertising, auto safety, and the functioning of governmental consumer protective agencies.

For a number of years, the actions and stands of the consumer testing organizations did not make much headway with legislators. One reason was that the country had not yet solved its "level of production" problems, and no legislator wanted to do anything to hinder sales of anything, and thereby slow down production. As the country moved to the solution of its production problems, legislators began to pay more attention to the voice of the consumer. In the fifties, Senators Estes Kefauver, Paul Douglas, Philip Hart, Warren Magnuson, and Abraham Ribicoff and Representative Wright Patman put consumer-oriented legislation into the hopper in unprecedented volume.

In the 1960's, the consumer movement came into its own. President Kennedy formed a Consumer Advisory Council and attached it to the Council of Economic Advisors. The council gave consumers a direct link to the White House. This led, under Johnson, to the appointment of a special presidential assistant for consumer affairs in the President's Committee on Consumer Interests. One result was the establishment of liaison between about 32 voluntary consumer organizations and the President's Committee. In a message to Congress in 1964, President Johnson said, "We cannot rest content until [the consumer] is in the front row, not displacing the interest of the producer, yet gaining rank and representation with that interest."

In the late 1960's, the Consumer Federation of America was formed as a coordinating organization for the efforts of consumer, labor, and agricultural, rural electrification, and purchasing cooperatives in promoting a consumer program in Congress. In 1969, President Nixon climbed aboard the consumerism bandwagon. He kept the position of special assistant for consumer affairs and sent Congress a "consumer bill of rights."

Meanwhile much consumer legislation had been passed. There is the Federal Insecticide, Fungicide, and Pesticide Amendment of 1964; National Traffic and Motor Vehicle Safety Act of 1966; Fair Packaging and Labeling Act of 1966; Wholesome Meat Act of 1967; Consumer Credit Protection Act of 1968; Truth and Lending Act of 1968; Child Protection and Toy Act of 1969; and the health hazard warning on cigarette packages (1968).

With all this legislation, why can food, drug, and cosmetics producers turn out the harmful, unwholesome, or useless products that still are being put on the market? An answer is that the laws themselves are not enough; strict enforcement is necessary. And it is in the realm of enforcement that the federal agencies fail the citizens they are supposed to serve. Also, no sooner is a law passed than lobbyists are on Capitol Hill pressuring congressmen to pass amending legislation that riddles the law with loopholes.

Political Action

It is a characteristic of most people that they can become politically aware and active if they feel personally harmed by some action or if a leader arouses their political awareness. They remain active until they achieve the goal that aroused them; then they become inactive. The lobbyists and politicians never rest because politics is their business. To counter their efforts, you must be constantly alert and active concerning the causes you are interested in. This is easier said than done. Yet each citizen can be very effective politically if he or she tries. You can join a consumers group, such as Consumers Union. Your dues will support their activities and they will listen to what you have to say on consumer matters connected with the problem of body pollution. They have their own lobbyists in Washington; they will be lobbying for you. Then, you can write to your representative and senators. Most people feel that this is futile, but those who know Washington know that letters from constituents are taken very seriously by congressmen. Of course, they receive too many letters to read each one; but their assistants do read the letters and answer them. True, the answer may be a form letter, but the contents of your letter were noted and tabulated before the reply was sent to you. Enough letters on a particular subject will make even the weakest congressman stand up to the lobbyists. Make it a habit to write a couple of letters every week. There is enough in this book alone on the subject of body pollution to keep you writing for years. How about starting right now by writing your congressmen that the Food and Drug Administration needs a shakeup, and why.

Economic Action

Economic action can be very effective. In a way, it is what the whole matter of the consumer versus the profit-hungry food processor or drug and cosmetic manufacturer is all about. If one of these producers finds that his polluted product is not selling, he will stop putting it on the market. After all, the only reason that adulterated and harmful food, drugs, and cosmetics are sold is to make money.

Again, we urge you to join some kind of consumer product-testing group, so that you can learn what you are buying. With knowledge of the products on the market, you certainly won't buy those that will harm you or are a waste of money.

You can be effective on the local level, too. Tell the merchants you deal with that you won't buy from them if they continue to sell products you know to be of a body-polluting nature. If you deal with a supermarket, get some friends together and picket the store. The manager will quickly listen to your complaints, and the supermarket's buyers will eventually hear about them.

Social Action

One of the most effective kinds of action is social. It is the kind that is taken by individuals upon seeing their friends, coworkers, or neighbors doing something that needs doing. Much of the work done to clean up the environment has been done by groups of individuals who formed because they felt a common need to do something. Simply setting a good example can be very effective. It could work this way:

If you have a lawn or garden, stop using pesticides and buy some black-light insect traps. Not only put them out, tell your neighbors about them and show how effective they are. A very large number of Americans are ecologically aware today. The insect trap idea could catch on. This would mean less pesticide draining into streams, rivers, and lakes, and less contamination of your drinking water.

The largest kind of green area in the United States is the house lawn. If you have one, show your neighbors how well it will grow with mulch instead of chemical fertilizer. Many neighbors will follow your lead. People really do want to cut down on pollution.

Legal Action

Another type of action you can take is legal action against the body polluters that you come up against every day when you buy and eat food. There are several ways to do this. If your pocket can afford it, you may take your complaint about a kind of food or cosmetic to a lawyer and let him handle the matter from there as a lawsuit. Very few of us are likely to do this. Instead, you can support one of the many organizations that employ legal staffs for the furtherance of consumers' rights and for the defense of the environment. One such organization is the Sierra Club, another is the Environmental Defense Fund, and there are others you can find if you ask environmentalists or consumer groups. The legal work is done by the organizations' legal staffs for you. All you have to do is help out financially through membership or a modest contribution. It was legal action by environmentalist groups that eventually led to the banning of DDT.

Most states and many local communities have consumer fraud divisions. By bringing your complaint to one of these, you can have legal action taken for you. You do not have to become ill from an adulterated food, for example, in order to take legal action against the processor. All you need to do is to show that the food violates some part of the Federal Food, Drug, and Cosmetic Act, the Wholesome Meat Act, or some other law or governmental regulation.

Section 402,b,1 of the Federal Food, Drug, and Cosmetic Act says: "A substance recognized as being a valuable constituent of food must not be omitted or abstracted in whole or in part . . ." Why not complain to a consumer fraud department, pointing out that enforcement of this part of the Act makes refined sugar and wheat minus wheat germ unlawful.

Section 402,b,2 says: ". . . nor may any substance be substituted for the food in whole or in part." Enforcement of this section would put an end to "enrichment" and "fortification" of foods that have had nutrients removed.

You can find in consumer protection laws dozens of other grounds for legal action to defend yourself against body pollution.

Immediate Personal Action

While engaging in the social, political, and economic actions that we have discussed, every person can take immediate personal action to lessen the effects of the body-polluting environment in which he lives.

Cleansing the Body

Since you are continually taking into your body dozens of food additives, it makes sense to cleanse your body of these poisons every once in a while. One way in which you can do this is to make use of the techniques of *fasting*.

Fasting is a very old health measure. People used fasting as a therapeutic measure since the beginning of civilization. Fasting is a total or partial abstinence from food or water or both for any length of time, but usually more than a day. Fasting may be selective; one can abstain from a particular type of food or a combination of foods. There are fruit fasts, milk fasts, meat fasts, water fasts, vegetable fasts, and so on. The most common type of fast is total abstinence from all foods, but not from water.

Most people who undertake a fast know very little if anything about how fasting should be done. As a result, they suffer from unnecessary side effects of going without food for a relatively long period.

Although fasting is a valuable body-cleansing action, it is not a cure for any disease or ailment. Fasting allows the body to bring into play the full range and scope of its natural self-healing, self-rejuvenating, and self-repairing functions. Fasting gives your body a rest from the large number of physiological processes connected with digestion and the elimination of food wastes. It allows the body to become 100 per cent efficient in healing itself. This is why fasting can be a rapid and safe way of regaining health or of putting oneself in tip-top physical condition.

Fasting gives overworked and overburdened internal organs and tissues rest and time for repair and rejuvenation. It exhilarates the internal power and vitality of all bodily systems to rid themselves of toxic matter and other poisons that have accumulated in the body for a long time, usually for years. Thus, fasting promotes the elimination of inorganic chemical accumulations and other toxic matter which cannot be flushed from the body in the normal course of its functioning.

After a fast, you will find that all of your organs function better, which means that they are in better condition. Digestion, assimilation, and elimination will be improved. You will find that your senses, except sight, will be sharper and raised to a much higher than normal level of efficiency during and after a fast.

Fasting improves circulation and promotes vigor, endurance, strength, and stamina. In short, fasting renovates, revivifies, and purifies each one of the billions of cells that make up your body.

Fasting is natural among wild animals that are ill, although, of course, they do not do so as the result of any thought-out therapeutic action, but rather as an instinctual act. Intelligent persons in early civilizations made therapeutic use of fasting. The first of these were the early Greeks. In ancient times, many priests were priest-physicians, and people came to temples of worship to be healed. One way that these priest physicians persuaded some of their patients to fast was to state that the fast was the will of the gods. Eventually, there came to be religious fast days. These have persisted to our times. In the Roman Catholic religion there is Lent (a meat fast), Ember Days, and certain Vigils as fast days. In the Jewish religion, there is Yom Kippur; and in Mohammedanism, there are 30 days a year of total or partial fasting. It is a shame that but few modern believers in these religions adhere strictly to the fasting practices.

In ancient Greece, both Plato and Aristotle fasted many times in their lives. Pythagoras fasted for 40 days before taking his examination at the University of Alexandria. Ancient Egyptian writings refer to fasting as a remedy for syphilis and other diseases. The famous Greek physician Hippocrates prescribed fasting for many serious illnesses. The physicians Asclepiades and Thessalus practiced fasting. The philosopher Celsus fasted to treat his jaundice and epilepsy. The great Arabian physician Avicenna prescribed fasting for all ailments. The Greek biographer Plutarch wrote, "Instead of using medicine, better fast a day." Throughout history, men of science and medicine have practiced, spoken for, and written about the benefits of fasting.

What Happens When You Fast

If you abstain from food for any length of time, certain changes in the functions, chemical reactions, and life processes of cells and tissues take place in your body. It is these changes that give fasting its therapeutic properties.

One of the physiological effects of fasting is rejuvenation of the cells that make up the tissues of the body. The cells have an opportunity to rid themselves of accumulated waste matter and put themselves into a completely healthy state. Fasting also increases the metabolic rate. This was shown by Drs. Carlson and Kunde, of the Department of Physiology in the University of Chicago. After they put a 40-year-old man on a 14-day fast, his tissues were in the same physiological condition as those of a 17-year-old youth. That is, his tissues were rejuvenated.

A process that is effected by fasting is autolysis. This word means "self-digestion" and refers to digestion by enzymes of materials already within an organism. In the human body, during a fast, autolysis digests stored fats and useless cells in tissues.

During a fast, there is a redistribution of nutrients, the surpluses and nonvital nutrients being digested and utilized first.

Fasting increases the body's assimilative powers significantly. The iron and other nutrients stored in the tissues are taken up by the blood and used. This improves the condition of the blood, a situation that may account partially for the reduction in tooth decay after a fast. During the fast, swollen, inflamed, and bleeding gums are restored to normal. These gum conditions are a contributing factor to tooth decay. Of course, the obvious reason that tooth decay is lessened during a fast is that there is no food in the spaces between the teeth—food that nourishes tooth-decay bacteria.

Fasting may correct difficulties of assimilation. People who are chronically underweight despite a large food intake often gain weight to the normal level after regaining the weight lost during a fast. Some overweight people lose a large amount of weight during a fast, then regain weight only up to their normal level and not above it as they had done in the past. Fasting, then, can help both those who assimilate too much and those who assimilate too little.

A summary of the ways in which fasting can help you to attain improved health are:

1. Produces rejuvenation of tissues.
2. Induces autolysis.
3. Improves assimilation and elimination.
4. Allows the organs a physiological rest.
5. Increases acuteness of the senses (except eyesight).
6. Speeds up the healing processes for certain bodily ailments.

Individuals who have been undergoing a long treatment with drugs for certain chronic illnesses benefit by fasting, as the accumulated drugs are eliminated from their bodies.

Your body has a considerable amount of stored food in the form of fat and other food elements. From the beginning of a fast, the body begins to nourish itself on the stored reserves. The body loses weight in the form of fat, muscle tissue, blood plasma, and water. As long as the reserves exist, the fast is a healthy one. When the reserves are used up, tissues of vital organs begin to be used up in the autolytic processes. The person fasting is then in danger, and continued fasting can lead to death.

How to Fast

Fasting begins with abstinence from food and ends when the body's food reserves are used up. There are certain very definite signs that appear when the reserves are used up. There is (1) a return of hunger and (2) a clearing of the coating on the tongue. The edges and tip of the tongue clear first; the remainder of the tongue clears quickly thereafter. In addition to these two main signs, the foul breath and bad taste in the mouth, which accompany fasting, disappear. Still another sign warning you to end your fast is a sharp drop in body temperature, an onset of chilling. If the pulse and temperature have become abnormal, they return to normal. Even if the person fasting wishes to continue his fast, he should break it when the first of the aforementioned signs appear. Even if the second of the two main signs does not appear—if the tongue does not clear —the fast should be broken. Failure to understand the end-of-fast signs can make the difference between fasting and starving. Once the autolysis of the vital organs begins, fasting has ended and starvation has begun.

Since the length of a fast depends on each individual's reserve supply, and you cannot know how long your reserve will last, you should not set an arbitrary length of fasting time. Just begin the fast and watch for the end-of-fast signs.

You will notice some discomforts during the initial stages of the fast. On the first day, a very strong desire for food will be present by afternoon or early evening. On the second day the desire will increase, but by the third day, this craving will abate. On the fourth or fifth day, hunger will disappear. During the first few days after your hunger has worn off, you may feel a strong repugnance for food. Any time in the first few days of the fast, your tongue probably will become coated and your breath foul. You may experience nausea and vomiting. Later in the fast your pulse may slow and become erratic. If the pulse remains erratic for more than a day, you should end your fast.

Your strength will wane all during the fast. You may feel very weak during the first few days, then feel stronger, but your strength will gradually become less and less. If you become so weak that you faint or are unable to walk, end your fast.

It is not possible to say how quickly you will lose weight; the rate of loss depends on how big and how heavy you are, as well as whether your weight is mostly muscle or fat. You should not let the fast continue to the point of extreme emaciation. Fat people have DDT stored in their fat, and as the fat is used up in autolysis, the DDT will be released into the bloodstream, and nausea may result.

During your fast, sexual desire will diminish greatly or entirely disappear. This is not cause for alarm; the sexual urge will return after the fast has ended.

If your fast lasts more than a couple of days, you must drink water. Otherwise, extreme dehydration will take place and death will follow. It is not necessary to drink large quantities of water. A tumbler of water every few hours, or five times a day, is sufficient. If hot weather or low humidity causes you to thirst for more water, drink it.

Ending the Fast

When you have noted the end-of-fast signs, break your fast by taking liquid nourishment: fruit juices and vegetable juices. Also, bouillon. Milk may be difficult to keep down. Take small amounts of nourishment at first, and take them slowly. During the fast the size of your stomach and intestines shrink, and you must not try to stretch them too suddenly. The liquids should be at room temperature or near it, not hot or cold.

On the first day, take half a glass of liquid nourishment every hour, or (after the first half-glass) one glassful every two hours. The juice diet should be continued for the length of time shown in the following table:

Length of fast	Length of juice diet
1–3 days	1 day
4–8 "	2 days
9–15 "	3 "
16–24 "	4 "
25–35 "	5 "
over 35 "	6 "

Following the juice diet, eat in moderation. Do not try to hurry back to a normal amount of daily food.

Do not think that because you have had a successful fast you are now immune to illness or disease. The only insurance you have to keep ailments out of your life is to live properly. Try to control your eating habits in order to preserve your good health. So, understand fasting for what it is: a means of promoting the remedy of illness and the creation of health. It is not a method of maintaining health.

Raw Juice Therapy

Another method, in addition to fasting, of cleansing the body internally is raw food juice therapy.

Plants are the basis of all foods for human beings. Man eats plants or he eats animals that eat plants. Plant juices are the lifeblood of plants and contain vital enzymes and digestive factors so essential to maintaining a healthy body. The juices exhibit valuable therapeutic properties. They do not have the toxic effect of drugs. Raw plant juices can sometimes eliminate and often prevent many chronic and degenerative diseases.

Raw juices require no digestion as compared with cooked foods. The juices remain in the stomach a very short time and are more thoroughly assimilated than any other foodstuffs. They are absorbed directly into the blood. The vitamins and minerals are unchanged by heating as is the case with cooked foods.

Why Juices?

You may wonder why we recommend the juices instead of the whole vegetables or fruits. Why not simply eat raw fruits and vegetables? The answer is that to get as much juice as you need, you would have to eat more than it is possible for you to put into your stomach at one time. Even if you gorged yourself, your stomach could not digest the amount of bulk, or roughage, that you would put into your stomach. Also, juicing and pulverizing food breaks it down more thoroughly than chewing.

Fruit juices are cleansers of the human system. Vegetable juices build and regenerate the human system. A diet which is properly balanced and uses a large amount of raw food juices can only help to prolong life and prevent illness. Cooking destroys most of the vitamins available in raw food juice. A pint or more of fresh raw juice will aid in keeping a person in good overall condition, but any therapeutic effect cannot be obtained overnight or even within a very short time. A minimum of six weeks or longer is needed for your body to use the elements in raw juices to rebuild diseased or worn out tissue.

The body's eliminative processes begin to detoxify your body within a few hours of drinking raw juices. As the blood becomes more alkaline because of the juices, toxins which have saturated the cells are dissolved and enter the bloodstream to be carried off via the regular excretory channels. Some bowel discomfort may, indeed usually will, appear during the first few weeks of juice therapy. You should not take this discomfort to mean that juices should no longer be ingested.

Blood cells are replaced after 14 days. If you have plenty of vegetable juices, your new cells will be healthier. Raw juices have a normalizing effect on intestinal flora and the juice has an absorbing effect on the intestinal mucous membrane.

Besides the faithful and continued taking of raw juices you must have a knowledge of the cleansing and healing properties of each type of raw juice. For instance, carrot juice is one of the richest sources of vitamin A and also contains valuable amounts of vitamins C, K, and riboflavin. It assists a sluggish appetite and aids digestion and it can improve and help maintain the bony structure of the teeth. Carrot juice also gives you energy that combats fatigue. It also helps your body resist infection and is good for your nervous system.

General Rules

For general health, have an eight-ounce glass of apple or orange juice in the morning, an eight-ounce glass of carrot juice in the afternoon, and an eight-ounce glass of grapefruit juice before going to bed at night.

Apple juice a half hour after you rise in the morning assists the overall functioning of the body and promotes peristaltic activity of the intestines. Carrot juice, as we have noted, helps to keep the mucous membranes, cells, glands, bones, and walls of the arteries in a healthy condition. Grapefruit or celery juice before bed soothes, relaxes, and allows for a more sound sleep.

The Various Juices

The following detailed descriptions will give you a comprehensive look at the value of single and combined juices.

Raw Carrot Juice. In addition to the properties already stated for this juice, it is a blood-building agent, particularly when combined with lettuce and beet juices. Besides vitamins A, C, and K, and riboflavin, carrot juice also contains vitamins B and E. Carrot juice is the single most important juice you can drink because it combines well with any other juice and contains the most nutrients of any juice. Carrot juice enriches the quality of the milk of nursing mothers.

Apple Juice purges the system of impurities and tones the cells. It has a good supply of potassium, sodium, and phosphorus. It is an excellent kidney stimulant in addition to promoting intestinal activity.

Celery Juice is the most potent nerve tonic of any juice. It also contains beneficial amounts of potassium, calcium, phosphorus, and sodium. It helps to keep calcium in distribution, which aids arthritic conditions.

Carrot and Celery Juices combined are an excellent combination for cleansing the system and in combating acidosis, or excess acid in the system. This combination has all the beneficial properties of the two juices that make it up.

Carrot, Celery, and Parsley Juices give you the same beneficial nutrients as carrot and celery juice, but parsley, being very strong, does a very good job of cleansing the kidneys. It energizes the adrenal glands and has a powerful therapeutic effect on the nervous system. Parsley juice is so powerful that it should not be taken alone, but always in combination with carrot, celery, apple, or orange juice. An overdose of parsley juice will overstimulate the nervous system. Never drink more than an ounce of pure parsley juice.

Carrot and Beet Juices. The amount of iron in beet juice will provide the red blood corpuscles with the iron they need. The combination of carrot and beet juice contains a high percentage of phosphorus and sulfur and also potassium and other alkaline minerals. These added to the high vitamin A, which is in the carrot juice, make a stronger builder of blood cells.

Cucumber, Beet, Parsley, and Carrot Juices. If you add cucumber juice to carrot, beet, and parsley juices, you will have a cleansing potion for the liver, gall bladder, kidneys, and prostate and other sex glands.

Carrot and Cabbage Juice contains a large proportion of sulfur and chlorine and is high in iodine. This results in a cleanser for the mucous membrane of the intestine and stomach.

Many persons have found that gas pains occur shortly after drinking raw cabbage juice. If this happens to you, drink two 16-ounce glasses of carrot and spinach juice daily for two or three weeks. This will thoroughly clean out your intestinal tract.

Carrot and cabbage juice is a good source of vitamin C. It is beneficial for infections of the gums.

Boiling or dehydrating destroys most of the valuable vitamins in fruit and vegetable juices. One half pint of raw cabbage juice contains more organic food value than does two hundred pounds of cooked or canned cabbage.

Carrot and Radish Juice and Horseradish Sauce make a potent cleanser of abnormal mucus in the system. One half teaspoonful of fresh horseradish sauce should be taken twice a day between meals. If you feel you must mix something with the horseradish, do not use vinegar. Instead, add a teaspoonful of lemon juice, but do not dilute the horseradish further. Also, do not drink anything for at least half an hour before taking the horseradish. The sauce may cause you to tear copiously. This will aid in clearing mucus in the sinus cavities. This is a natural method of cleansing these head cavities.

Never drink raw radish juice undiluted; it is too strong. It should be combined with carrot juice which has a soothing and healing effect.

Lettuce Juice is loaded with iron and magnesium. Also, 38 per cent potassium, nearly 15 per cent calcium, 5 per cent iron, 6 per cent sulfur, 9 per cent phosphorus, 8 per cent silicon, some sodium, as well as trace elements.

Spinach Juice provides food for the entire digestive tract: the stomach, duodenum, and small and large intestines. Spinach juice is as good a method of cleansing the intestinal tract as one can find. By combining an equal amount of apple juice with spinach juice, you can correct the most aggravated case of constipation within a few days or weeks.

Raw spinach juice has proved to be effective in cases of pyorrhea. Bleeding gums and fibroid degeneration of the pulp of the teeth has become a common ailment due to the poor quality of the typical American diet with its emphasis on concentrated starches, fats, and poor food combinations.

Raw spinach juice contains a high percentage of oxalic acid which can combine with calcium, forming calcium oxalate, the material of which kidney stones are made. Therefore, spinach juice should be taken with caution and avoided by those suffering from kidney trouble.

Turnip Leaf Juice has the highest percentage of calcium found in any vegetable. This juice should be taken by anyone who has a calcium deficiency. The combination of carrot and dandelion juices with turnip leaf juice makes a tonic unmatched for strengthening the teeth and bones.

Turnip leaf juice is high in potassium, which makes it a good alkalizer, particularly when combined with celery and carrot juices.

Watercress Juice contains much sulfur, phosphorus, and chlorine, which make it acidic. For this reason, it should never be drunk alone, but should be combined with carrot or celery juice. Watercress juice is a strong intestinal cleanser.

Cucumber Juice has a diuretic action, that is, it promotes the flow of urine. By combining carrot juice with cucumber juice you will have a strong tonic for helping rheumatic ailments resulting from an excessive amount of uric acid in your system.

Dandelion Juice is beneficial in counteracting hyperacidity and in normalizing the alkalinity of the system. It is very rich in magnesium and also contains considerable amounts of calcium and sodium. A good tonic for spinal and other bone ailments is a combination of carrot and turnip juices added to raw dandelion juice.

Fennel Juice has qualities similar to celery juice. It is very beneficial for the entire optic system and contains nearly all of the essential vitamins and minerals.

Tomato Juice is also rich in vitamins and minerals and helps to neutralize an excessively acid condition. If you drink tomato juice during the same meal in which you eat acid-forming foods such as some carbohydrates, you will neutralize the tomato juice. Therefore, if you want the alkalizing effect of tomato juice, do not drink it along with eating the acid-forming foods.

Onion and Garlic Juices have an odor which some people consider to be unpleasant. These juices provide the system with a strong tonic that helps nervousness, insomnia, and rheumatism and is a good blood purifier. It also helps to kill harmful bacteria in the nose and throat.

Carrot and Coconut Juices provide the system with ample amounts of calcium, magnesium, and iron, and help to build a strong body.

Grapefruit, Cabbage, and Coconut Juices contain chlorine and sulfur. This combination is an excellent diuretic and is good for cleansing the mucous membranes of the stomach and intestinal tract. It also is a natural antiseptic.

Carrot, Apple, and Beet Juices provide a very good tonic rich in minerals and valuable in cases of constipation, tired blood, obesity, and general fatigue.

Carrot, Spinach, and Orange Juices are good for the entire digestive tract, the stomach, duodenum, and intestines.

Celery, Tomato, and Radish Juices are strong natural antiseptics. They protect your system against infection and aid in obesity, catarrh, constipation, and nerve disorders.

Pineapple Juice contains a digestive enzyme called papain. It is rich in chlorine which helps to digest proteins.

Orange Juice is a good cleanser of the intestinal tract and a blood purifier. It is an excellent alkalizer and is rich in vitamin C.

Grapefruit Juice is much like orange juice, being a good alkalizer, and it is rich in fruit acids (which have an alkaline reaction in the digestive tract) and sugars.

Blueberry and Huckleberry Juices act as a natural astringent, antiseptic, and blood purifier. Persons suffering from acidosis, menstruation disorders, and high blood pressure should drink an eight-ounce glass twice daily.

Strawberry, Cherry, Prune, and Date Juices provide an instant booster for the sluggish system, including sluggish skin, poor complexion, sore eyes, and quinsy.

The foregoing raw juice combinations should give you an idea of the possibilities inherent in these natural healing and health-maintaining juices. In a book of this scope we have not been able to include the exact amounts of each juice that should go into each juice combination. We have given these in detail in another book, *The Complete Handbook of Nutrition*, by Gary and Steve Null. This book also contains tables telling which nutritional deficiencies can be made up by various raw juice combinations.

Improved Diet

Food Combining

To maintain a healthy eating program, there are two basic rules that one must follow. The first is to understand exactly which foods contain what food values and, secondly, how one should combine foods in order to fully utilize, digest and assimilate them. The following chapter explains the proper combination in which foods should be eaten.

The amount of each food eaten depends upon the individual. It is rather obvious that most Americans are not yet ready to discipline themselves to eating all of the right foods in the proper combinations all of the time. We realize that changing the American diet and methods of eating will take years, but if we show what constitutes the ultimate method, it may help those few who wish to make the change in diet gradually.

How to Eat Fruits

Fruits undergo little or no digestion in the mouth and stomach and are, as a rule, quickly passed into the inestine, where they undergo the little digestion they require. Since fruits pass into the intestine so readily, it is better not to eat them between meals in order to afford the intestine a rest after it has finished digesting the last-eaten meal.

A very healthy and tasty meal may be made of fruits as follows:

Grapefruit, orange, apple, pineapple, lettuce, celery, four ounces of cottage cheese or four ounces of nuts or a greater amount of avocado.

How to Eat Starch

We suggest that the starch meal should be eaten at noon. Starches should be eaten dry and should be thoroughly chewed and insalivated before swallowing. Acidic foods should not be eaten with the starch meal. The following are three sample starch meals. We suggest that the salad be a small one.

Vegetable salad	Vegetable salad	Vegetable salad
Turnip greens	Spinach	String beans
Yellow squash	String beans	Mashed rutabaga
Chestnuts	Coconut	Irish potatoes

How to Eat Proteins

The foods that combine best with proteins of all types are the nonstarchy and succulent vegetables. It is suggested that the protein meal be eaten in the evening. Acid foods, oils, and oily dressings should be kept to a minimum with protein meals. The following are three sample protein meals.

Vegetable salad	Vegetable salad	Vegetable salad
Green squash	Chard	Collards
Spinach	Yellow squash	Yellow squash
Nuts	Fowl	Lean meat

Eating Schedule for a Week

We wish to stress that all the menus given in this book are intended merely as guides to the reader to assist him to understand the principles of food combining and to enable him to work out his own menus.

The following two weekly schedules are designed to demonstrate the proper way to combine foods at different seasons of the year. The first week's schedule covers foods available in spring and summer. The second week's schedule covers foods available in fall and winter. Use these merely as guides and learn to prepare your own menus. The proteins are only suggestions and may be changed to suit your taste.

SPRING AND SUMMER MENUS

BREAKFAST	LUNCH	DINNER
	Sunday	
Watermelon	Vegetable salad	Vegetable salad
	Chard	String beans
	Yellow squash	Okra
	Potatoes	Lean meat
	Monday	
Peaches	Vegetable salad	Vegetable salad
Cherries	Beet greens	Spinach
Apricots	Carrots	Cabbage
	Baked beans	Fowl
	Tuesday	
Cantaloupes	Vegetable salad	Vegetable salad
	Okra	Broccoli
	Green squash	Fresh corn
	Jerusalem artichoke	Eggs
	Wednesday	
Berries with Cream	Vegetable salad	Vegetable salad
(no sugar)	Cauliflower	Green squash
	Okra	Turnip greens
	Brown rice	Lean meat

Thursday

Nectarines	Vegetable salad	Vegetable salad
Apricots	Green cabbage	Beet greens
Plums	Carrots	String beans
	Sweet potatoes	Fowl

Friday

Watermelon	Vegetable salad	Vegetable salad
	Baked eggplant	Yellow
	Chard	Spinach
	Whole wheat bread	Fish

Saturday

Bananas	Vegetable salad	Vegetable salad
Cherries	Green beans	Broccoli
Glass of sour milk	Okra	Soy sprouts
	Irish potatoes	Lean meat

FALL AND WINTER MENUS

BREAKFAST	LUNCH	DINNER

Sunday

Grapes	Vegetable salad	Vegetable salad
Bananas	Chinese cabbage	Spinach
Dates	Asparagus	Yellow squash
	Baked caladium roots	Fish

Monday

Persimmons	Vegetable salad	Vegetable salad
Pears	Kale	Brussels sprouts
Grapes	Cauliflower	String beans
	Yams	Fowl

Tuesday

Apples	Vegetable salad	Vegetable salad
Grapes	Turnip	Yellow squash
Dried figs	Okra	Lean meat
	Brown rice	Kale

Wednesday

Pears	Vegetable salad	Vegetable salad
Persimmons	Broccoli	Okra
Banana	String beans	Spinach
Glass of sour milk	Irish potatoes	Fish

Thursday

Papaya	Vegetable salad	Vegetable salad
Orange	Green squash	Red cabbage
	Parsnips	String beans
	Whole grain bread	Fowl

Friday

Persimmons	Vegetable salad	Vegetable salad
Grapes	Carrots	Chard
Dates	Spinach	Yellow squash
	Steamed caladium roots	Cheese (Swiss, American, and Cheddar, etc.)

Saturday

Grapefruit	Vegetable salad	Vegetable salad
	Fresh peas	Spinach
	Kale	Steamed onions
	Coconut	Lamb chops

Right and Wrong Combinations

To understand fully what combinations of foodstuffs you can digest, it will be necessary to consider, one by one, the possible combinations and analyze these in their relation to the facts of digestion.

Acid-Starch Combinations

A weak acid will destroy ptyalin, the component of saliva that digests starch in the mouth. Starch not digested in the mouth will be digested in other parts of the digestive system. Yet, it would be better to have starch digestion take place in the mouth. Therefore, it is better not to eat acid foods such as tomatoes, berries, oranges, grapefruits, lemons, limes, pineapples, sour apples, sour grapes, at the same times you are eating starch.

Protein-Starch Combinations

Proteins are digested best in an acid medium. Therefore, it is unwise to eat both starch and protein at the same time; the starch needs an alkaline medium and the protein an acid medium, and both cannot be provided at the same time in the part of the digestive system. For these reasons, we recommend the eating of starches and proteins at separate meals. This means that cereals, bread, potatoes, and other starchy foods should not be eaten at the same time you eat meats, eggs, cheese, and other protein foods.

Protein-Protein Combinations

Not all proteins are of the same quality, because each protein is made up of a different combination of amino acids. This means that the body digests different protein foods differently. Therefore, it is unwise to mix certain proteins. One type of protein per meal will result in greater efficiency of digestion.

We do not recommend eating at the same meal meat and eggs, meat and nuts, meat and cheese, eggs and milk, eggs and nuts, cheese and nuts, milk and nuts, and other combinations of these protein foods. Our recommendation is: Eat but one concentrated protein food per meal.

Protein-Acid Combinations

Although protein is digested in an acid medium, it is the body that should provide the acid. Eating acid foods along with protein can provide too much acid. Therefore we recommend eating proteins and acid foods at separate meals.

Nuts or cheese eaten with acid fruits do not constitute an ideal combination, but we make exception to the foregoing rule in the case of these two articles of food. Nuts and cheese, containing considerable oil and fat (cream), are about the only exceptions to the rule that when acids are eaten with protein, putrefaction occurs. These foods do not decompose as quickly as other protein when they are not immediately digested. Furthermore, acids do not delay the digestion of nuts and cheese, because these foods contain enough fat to inhibit gastric secretion for a longer time than do acids.

Fat-Protein Combinations

Fat exerts an inhibiting influence on the secretion of gastric juice. The inhibiting effect may last two or more hours. This means that when protein is eaten, fat should not be eaten at the same meal. In other words, such foods as cream, butter, various kinds of oils, gravies, meat fats should not be eaten at the same meal with nuts, cheese, eggs, and flesh. Thus, our recommendation is: Eat fats and proteins at separate meals.

We recommend the eating of raw green vegetables to counteract the inhibiting effect of fat.

Sugar-Protein Combinations

All sugars—commercial (refined) sugars, syrups, sweet fruits, and even honey—hinder protein digestion. Sugars are digested in the intestine. If eaten alone, they move quickly into the intestine. If eaten with other foods, their progress into the intestine is slowed. As a result, the sugars undergo fermentation in the stomach. Therefore, our recommendation is: Eat sugars and proteins at separate meals.

Sugar-Starch Combinations

The digestion of starch begins in the mouth and may continue in the stomach. Sugars, as we have seen, are digested in the small intestine, and the delay of this intestinal digestion may result in fermentation. In order that the digestion of sugar proceed as rapidly as possible, it is unwise to eat sugar and starch at the same time. Therefore we recommend: Eat starches and sugars at separate meals.

With the foregoing recommendations in mind, you can combine foods in ways that will best expedite their digestion, and therefore enable you to eat in the most healthful manner.

Know What You
Are Buying:
Handbook of Additives

If you know anything about food additives, it is only natural and reasonable to worry about what you are eating. Since the present laws require a considerable amount of truth in revealing just what is contained in packaged foods, you can know what additives are in a particular kind of food by reading the label on the package. However, there is a difference between reading the words on the package and really knowing what they mean in terms of the healthfulness or harmfulness of the additive. The following is a short handbook of food additives, listing and explaining the most common ones. Since there are thousands of them, the list must necessarily be incomplete. For the reader who is interested in a more complete compilation of food additives, we suggest *A Consumer's Dictionary of Food Additives*, by Ruth Winter (Crown Publishers, New York). This work lists thousands of additives and describes them in detail.

Agar-agar (or Japanese isinglass) Used as a stabilizer and thickener. It is transparent, tasteless, and odorless. Agar-agar is obtained from several kinds of seaweeds that grow in the Pacific and Indian Oceans and in the Sea of Japan. It is used in ice cream, ices, frozen custard, sherbet, beverages, jellies and preserves, meringue, baked goods, icings, candied sweet potatoes, and confections; may be used as a substitute for gelatin; and may be a thickener in milk and cream. Nontoxic. GRAS°

Ascorbic acid (Vitamin C) The antiscurvy vitamin; it is essential for healthy bones, teeth, and blood vessels. It also is a preventive and remedy for the common cold. Ascorbic acid is believed by some authorities to clear cholesterol deposits from the arteries. It is added to fruit juices, frozen and concentrated fruit drinks, orange and lemonade, and carbonated drinks. It is used as an antioxidant and preservative in frozen fruits (particularly peaches), frozen fish dips, dry milk solids, fluid milk, beer and ale, apple juice, candy, soft drinks, artificially sweetened jellies and preserves, canned mushrooms, and flavoring oils. It is put into the pickling liquid in which beef and pork are cured; also used in packing pulverized, cured, and cooked meat products. Ascorbic acid may be toxic when ingested along with sodium salicylate, sodium nitrate, theobromine sodium salicylate, and methenamine; also barbiturates.

Benzaldehyde (or benzoic aldehyde) An essential oil derived from almonds or made synthetically. Occurs naturally in almonds, cassia bark, bitter oil, cajeput oil, tea, raspberries, cherries. It is used in apricot, brandy, rum, peach, liquor, cherry, berry, butter, coconut, pistachio, almond, pecan, vanilla, and spice flavorings. Also in ice cream, candy, ices, beverages, cordials, baked goods, and chewing gum. It may cause a skin rash and it is narcotic in high concentrations. Large amounts produce convulsions and central nervous system depression. The fatal dose is approximately two ounces. GRAS

Butylated hydroxyanisole (BHA) A white or slightly yellow waxy solid. It is a preservative and antioxidant widely used in breakfast cereals, baked goods, potato flakes, sweet potato flakes, dry mixes for desserts and beverages, shortenings, lard,

---

° GRAS: *Generally Recognized As Safe* list of additives certified by the Food and Drug Administration.

dry yeast, soup bases, chewing gum, ices, glacéed fruits, beverages, and unsmoked dry sausage. Allowed up to 50 parts per million (ppm) with BHT (*which see*) in dry cereals; 50 ppm in potato flakes; 1000 ppm in dry yeast; up to 0.02 per cent of fat and oil content of food. Some suspected harmful effects which the FDA is investigating.

Butylated hydroxytoluene (BHT) A white crystalline solid. It is an antioxidant used in white potato and sweet potato flakes and in dry breakfast cereals; a chewing gum base; and emulsion stabilizer for animal fats and shortenings containing animal fats. Also used as an antioxidant to retard rancidity in frozen fresh pork and freeze-dried meats in amounts up to 0.01 per cent of the fat content; allowed as 50 ppm in dry breakfast cereals and potato flakes; up to 200 ppm in emulsion stabilizers. Experiments with rats have indicated harmful effects. BHT is under investigation by the FDA, but is on its GRAS list. BHT is banned in foods in England.

Carrageenan chondrous extract (or simply carrageenan) A gluelike derivative of Irish moss having a seaweedlike odor and a salty taste. It is used as an emulsifier and stabilizer in chocolate products, chocolate milk, chocolate-flavored drinks, pressure-dispensed whipped cream, confections, syrups for frozen products, evaporated milk, cheese spreads, ice cream, sherbets, frozen custard, ices, French dressing, and artificially sweetened jellies and jams. Ammonium, calcium, sodium, and potassium salts of carrageenan are used in syrups, jellies, puddings, baked goods, and beverages. Also used in medicinal syrup for soothing mucous membrane irritation. Sodium carrageenan is in the FDA's list for study for mutagenic, teratogenic, reproductive, and subacute effects, but is on the GRAS list.

Citric acid A varied additive used in the United States for almost a century. It is a colorless or white crystalline solid, having a strong acid taste. It is found in plant and animal tissues and fluids, and is produced commercially from the fermentation of crude sugar, or by extraction from citrus fruits. Besides occurring naturally in citrus fruits, it is found in peaches and coffee beans. It is used to adjust the acid-alkaline balance of candies, jams, jellies, wines, fruit juices, canned fruit, carbonated beverages, frozen fruit, canned vegetables, sherbet, cheese spreads, frozen dairy products, confections, dried egg white, mayonnaise, salad dressing, canned figs, fruit butter, preserves, fresh beef blood. Citric acid is also used in curing meats, firming peppers, potatoes, tomatoes, and lima beans; and to prevent off-flavors in potato chips and French-fried potatoes. It imparts a fruit flavor to beverages (2500 ppm), candy (4300 ppm), chewing gum (3600 ppm), ice cream, and ices. Medicinally, it has been used to dissolve urinary bladder stones. Non-toxic. GRAS

Citrus Red No. 2 A dye used for coloring orange skins of oranges *not* intended for processing, and which meet minumum ripeness standards established by the laws of states in which the oranges are grown. Oranges colored with Citrus Red No. 2 must not bear more than 2 ppm, calculated on the weight of the whole fruit. The toxicity of Citrus Red No. 2 is not entirely determined. One constituent of the dye, 2-naphthol, if ingested in quantity can cause clouding of the eye lens, vomiting, kidney damage, and circulatory collapse. Application of this constituent to the skin can cause peeling and death if it is on a large area.

Dextrin (or British gum, starch gum) A white or yellow powder made from starch. Used as a foam stabilizer for beer (causing the foam to last longer), a diluting agent for pills and dry extracts; for thickening industrial dye pastes; in matches, explosives, and fireworks; in dry bandages; for preparing emulsions; and in polishing cereals. Non-toxic. GRAS

Diethylstilbestrol (DES, or stilbestrol) A synthetic estrogen fed to cattle and poultry (prior to the autumn of 1972) to fatten them. It is still allowed as pellets implanted in the necks of young poultry, but this use is under investigation. DES is a known carcinogen. In 1971, it was shown that daughters of women who had taken DES during pregnancy developed a rare form of cancer. Cattle fed DES were supposed to be taken off DES feed for a length of time that allowed the estrogen to be eliminated from the animals' bodies. However, tests showed residues of DES in refrigerated meat. Since there may be a lapse of two years between slaughter and sale of meat, diethylstilbestrol is still to be found in meat from cattle fed this hormone. The European Common Market, Sweden, and Italy have banned the use of DES in cattle.

Disodium guanylate A flavor intensifier. It is the disodium salt of 5'-guanylic acid, found throughout nature as a compound in the formation of RNA and DNA. It is obtained from certain kinds of mushrooms. It is not known to be toxic.

Disodium phosphate A sequestering agent. It is used in evaporated milk (up to 0.1 per cent of finished product); in macaroni and noodle products (0.5 to 1.0 per cent). It is used as an emulsifier in cheeses (3 per cent by weight). It has U.S. Department of Agriculture clearance for use in preventing cookout juices in cured pork shoulders and loins; cured, canned, and chopped hams; and bacon. Disodium phosphate is also used as a buffer in adjusting acidity of chocolate products, beverages, enriched farina, and sauces and toppings. Medicinally, it has uses as a cathartic, purgative, and in phosphorus deficiency treatment. It can irritate the skin and mucous membranes. GRAS

Ethylinediamine tetraacetate (EDTA) A sequestrant in carbonated beverages. It is used in cooked and canned crab meat to prevent formation of struvite crystals and to retain color of the meat. Also used in nonstandard dressings. It is on the FDA's list for possible harmful effects. EDTA may irritate the skin and mucous membranes, and may cause sensitization leading to asthma and allergic skin rashes.

FD and C colors (food, drug and cosmetic colors) These are color additives, which means that they are dyes, pigments, or other substances capable of coloring a food or a drug or cosmetic used anywhere in or on the human body. Legislation in 1938 required that all the additive colors be given numbers and that every batch be certified. Illnesses caused by some of the colors led to their being taken off the approved list. In 1959, the FDA approved the use of "lakes," which are the dyes mixed with calcium or aluminum hydrates. The result is an insoluble coloring material used in candies and to color egg shells. In 1960, a law was passed to require tests for determining the suitability of all colors prior to putting them on a permanent listing as acceptable. Orange B (150 ppm), for coloring sausage casings, and Citrus Red No. 2 (2 ppm) for dying orange skins are now permanently listed. Red No. 3, Yellow No. 5, Blue No. 3, and Red No. 40 are also on the permanent list without any restrictions. All other colors are on the temporary list. The World Health Organization lists as completely acceptable only Red No. 2, Yellow No. 5, Yellow No. 6, Blue No. 1, and Green No. 3.

Glycerides (monoglycerides, diglycerides, and monosodium glycerides of edible fats and oils) These are emulsifying and defoaming agents. They are used in bread and other baked goods to maintain softness (which they do by absorbing moisture from the air), in ices, ice cream, ice milk, milk, beverages, shortenings, lard, oleomargarine, chewing gum base, confections, chocolate, sweet chocolate, whipped toppings, and rendered animal fats. The diglycerides are on the FDA list for study as possible mutagenic, teratogenic, subacute, and reproductive effects, but are on the GRAS list.

Imitation flavor A flavor that contains any portion of materials that are not of natural origin. For example, if lemon flavoring is not made entirely from lemons, it must be labeled as imitation.

Inosinate A flavor intensifier made from inosinic acid. It is obtained from meat extract or dried sardines. Non-toxic.

Lecithin This substance is found in all living organisms, both plant and animal, as a constituent of nerve tissue and brain material. It is made up of choline, phosphoric acid, glycerine, and fatty acids in chemical combination. It is obtained commercially from eggs, corn, and soybeans. It is used as an antioxidant in breakfast cereals, candy, bread, rolls, buns, and other baked goods, sweet chocolate, and oleomargarine. *Hydroxylated lecithin* is a defoaming agent used in the production of yeast and beet sugar. Non-toxic.

Menthol A flavoring agent that occurs naturally in mints, raspberries, and betel nuts. Its chief source is oil of peppermint. It is used in caramel, fruit, butter, spearmint and peppermint flavorings in chewing gum, candy, ices, ice cream, baked goods, liqueurs, and beverages. It is used in perfumery, and medicinally in cough drops and nasal inhalers; also in cigarettes. In large doses it can cause severe abdominal pain, nausea, vomiting, vertigo, and coma. The lethal dose in rats is 2.0 grams per gram of body weight. GRAS

Monosodium glutamate (MSG) The monosodium salt of glutamic acid. It is found in soybeans, sugar beets, seaweed, and sea tangles. It is a flavor intensifier used in meats, soups, pickles, candies, and baked goods. MSG is believed to be the cause of the so-called "Chinese restaurant syndrome" in which diners suffer numbness, headaches, and chest pains after eating Chinese food containing MSG. Causes brain damage effects in rats, rabbits, chicks, and monkeys. Formerly was used in baby foods, but now is banned by the processors of these foods. Is on the FDA list for study as a possible cause of mutagenic, teratogenic, subacute, and reproductive effects, but is on the GRAS list.

Nitrate, potassium and sodium. Potassium nitrate is also known as saltpeter and niter. In concentrations up to 0.02 per cent, it is used as a color fixative in cured meats, in pickling brine (7 pounds per hundred gallons), and in chopped meat, such as hamburger (2.75 ounces per 100 pounds). Sodium nitrate, also called Chile saltpeter, is used as a color fixative in cured meats, frankfurters, bologna, bacon, uncooked smoked ham, poultry, wild game, meat spreads, Vienna sausages, potted meat, poultry, and spiced ham. Also used in baby foods. Nitrates combine with substances—secondary amines—found naturally in the stomach and in certain foods, producing powerful carcinogenic substances—nitrosamines. The combination of nitrates and certain stomach chemicals produce nitrites that have caused deaths of babies through the condition called methemoglobinemia, which cuts off oxygen from the brain. The FDA has given nitrates priority in testing for cancer-causing effects, and also mutagenic, teratogenic, subacute, and reproductive effects.

Nitrite, potassium and sodium. Potassium nitrite (up to 0.02 per cent) is used to fix color of cured meats. It reacts chemically with the myoglobin molecule of meats, giving them a red-blooded color, brings a tangy taste, and resists the growth of the spore of *Clostridium botulinum*, which is responsible for the almost always fatal botulism of spoiling meat. Nitrite is a color fixative in bacon, bologna, deviled ham, cured meat, potted meat, meat spreads, Vienna sausage, spiced ham, smoke-cured tuna, shad, and salmon. It is used as a cosmetic and in baby foods. As with nitrate, nitrite can combine with certain stomach and food chemicals—secondary amines—to form the cancer-causing agents, nitrosamines and nitrosamides. Deaths due to nitrites are known, and the FDA is giving nitrites the same priority testing that it is giving to nitrates. Meanwhile the

Department of Agriculture is holding use of nitrite to 200 ppm going into ready-to-eat meats, which lose some nitrite en route to the table.

Pectin (including low methoxyl pectin and sodium pectinate) Pectin is found in plant roots, stems, seeds, and fruits, where it acts as a cementing agent. It is a powder (coarse or fine) with a gluey taste, and almost odorless. The richest source of pectin is orange or lemon rind, which contains about 30 per cent. It is used as a thickener, bodying agent, or stabilizer for artificially sweetened beverages, ice cream, ice milk, water ices, fruit sherbets, syrups for frozen products; fruit jelly, preserves, jams to make up for a lack of natural pectin; French dressing. Medicinally, it is an anti-diarrheal agent. Nontoxic.

Potassium citrate A white or transparent powder, odorless, and having a cool salty taste. Used as a buffer in artificially sweetened jellies and preserves and in confections. Medicinally it is a gastric antacid and urinary alkalizer. GRAS

Sodium bisulfite (or sodium acid sulfite, or sodium hydrogen sulfite) A white powder used as a bleaching agent in ale, beer, wine, and other food products. The FDA is studying it for possible mutagenic effects, but it is on the GRAS list.

Sodium citrate White odorless crystals, powder, or granules, having a salty taste. Prevents "cream plug," the semisolid collection of fatty material at the top of a container of cream. Also prevents "feathering" when cream is put into coffee. It is used as an emulsifier in evaporated milk, ice cream, processed cheese; as a buffer for controlling acidity and preventing loss of carbonation in soft drinks; also used in fruit drinks, confections, jams, jellies, and preserves. GRAS

Sorbitol A white, crystalline powder with a sweet taste. It is found in berries, cherries, plums, pears, apples, seaweed, where it occurs due to the breakdown of dextrose. It is used as a sugar substitute for diabetics, but its safety for this use has not been proved. It is also used as a sequestrant in vegetable oils, a thickener in candy, a stabilizer and sweetener in frozen desserts used in special diets, as a humectant (retainer of moisture) and texturizing agent in soft drinks, shredded coconut, and dietetic fruits. The FDA has asked for further study of sorbitol.

The foregoing list was chosen from thousands of food additives because it is made up of those most frequently found on food packages. We hope that you will refer to it when reading the make-up of the food within the packages you buy. Knowing something about the additives in the packaged foods may make you feel better and safer. Or, it may make you feel worse—in which case you will not buy that particular food anymore and thereby cut down on your body pollution.

Bibliography

Clark, Linda, *Get Well Naturally*, Arco.
———, *Stay Young Longer*, Pyramid.
Harmer, Ruth Mulvey, *Unfit for Human Consumption*, Prentice-Hall.
Hunter, Beatrice Trum, *Consumer Beware*, Simon and Schuster.
———, *Gardening Without Poisons*, Berkley Medallion.
Longgood, William, *The Poisons in Your Food*, Pyramid.
Null, Gary, *Grow Your Own Food Organically*, Robert Speller & Sons.
Pendergast, Chuck, *Introduction to Organic Gardening*, Nash.
Ralph Nader Study Group, *Chemical Feast*, Grossman.
Rodale, J. I., *The Basic Book of Organic Gardening*, Ballantine.
———, and Staff, *Our Poisoned Earth and Sky*, Rodale Books.
———, *Vegetables and Fruit by the Organic Method*, Rodale Books.
Turner, F. Newman, *Fertility Farming*, Faber and Faber.
Sanford, David (ed.), *Hot Water on the Consumer*, Pitman.
Winter, Ruth, *Beware of the Food You Eat*, Crown.
Yudkin, John, *Sweet and Dangerous*, Peter H. Wyden.

Index

Abramson, Dr. Harold, 83
Acetate, 124, 125, 128
Acid-alkaline controls, 29
Acid foods, how to eat, 192, 193
Acidosis, 182
Acne, 99, 105
Additives, food, 27–34
    in bread, 38–39
    as cancer producing agents, 35–36
    combinations of, 33
    handbook of, 195–204
    harmfulness of, 29–30
    in margarine, 65
    psychochemical reactions to, 128–129
    reasons for, 28–29
Adriaenssens, Dr. L., 62
Advertisers, 72–73, 77, 81, 84
Advertising, fraudulent, 93
Agar-agar, 195–196
Agene (nitrogen trichloride), 31, 38
Alcoholics Anonymous, 131, 132, 133, 142
Alcoholism, 116, 131–142
    causes of, 134–138
    description of, 132–134
    nutritional treatment of, 138–140
    psychological aspect of, 131–132, 140–141
    social aspect of, 131, 132, 134
Alcoholism: The Nutritional Approach (Williams), 132
Alkaline-acid controls, 29
Alkaline chemicals, 53
Aminophenols, 75
Aniline dyes, 75

Antibiotic creams, 73
Antibiotics
    in animal feed, 40–41, 42–43, 44, 50, 53
    in fish, 48–49
Antioxidants, 47
Antiperspirants, 77–78
Antispoilants, 28
Appendicitis, 85
Apple juice, 181, 182, 185
Arsenic compounds, 44–45
Arthritis, 106–108
Artificial coloring, 28
Ascorbic acid (vitamin C), 196
Askey, Dr. E. V., 152
Aspirin, 81–82
Assimilation, correcting difficulties of, 176
Atherosclerosis, 87, 110
Atomic radiation as insect control, 14
Autolysis, 176

Baby foods, nitrates in, 24
Bailey, Dr. Lana, 22
Baking soda, 76
Balance of nature, upset of, 13–14, 19–20
Beef, 39–42
Beet juice, 182, 183, 185
Behrman, Dr. Howard, 73
Benzaldehyde, 57, 196
Benzoic acid, 65
Benzoic aldehyde, 196
BHA (butylated hydroxyanisole), 196–197

207

BHT (butylated hydroxytoluene), 197
Bicknell, Dr. Franklin, 40–41, 64, 65, 107
Biochemical individuality, 136–137
Biskind, Dr. Morton S., 3–4
Bleaching flour, 38
Blood sugar, 122–125, 126
Blueberry juice, 186
Bone diseases, 106–109
Boric acid, 83–84
Botanicals, 14
Brain, 122–123, 124–128
Brannan, Charles F., 12
Bread, 37–39
Bromelin, 42
Bryan, Dr. George T., 66
Butter, 53
Butter Yellow, 31

Cabbage juice, 183, 185
  for ulcer patients, 113–114
Calcium, 98, 104, 108–109, 111, 135, 184
Calcium carbonate, 109
Calcium chloride, 52
Calcium gluconate, 109
Calcium lactate, 109, 111
Calcium salts, 29, 109
Calcium silicate, 29
Campbell, Dr. Douglas Gordon, 12
Cancer, 8, 24–25, 30, 35–36, 66, 112. See also Carcinogens
Carbamates, 7
Carbohydrates, 123
Carbon, polymerized, 35
Carcinogens, 35–36, 45, 51, 53, 54, 65, 66, 112, 199, 202
Caries, 76, 98, 103–105
Carlson, Dr., 175
Carotene, 53
Carrageenan, 52, 197
Carrot juice, 181, 182, 183, 185
Catalase, 30
Cataracts, 88, 101

Cattle-raising, 39–42
Cavities. See Caries
Celery juice, 181, 182, 185–186
Chapman, R. A., 32
Cheeses, 53
Cherry juice, 186
Chickens. See Poultry raising
Chlorinated hydrocarbons, 7, 8, 12. See also DDT
Chlorine, 49
Chlorine dioxide, 38
Cholesterol, 110–111
Cirrhosis of liver, 116
Citric acid, 29, 65, 197–198
Citric acid cycle, 125
Citrus Red No. 2 dye, 198, 200
Coal tar derivatives, 31, 36, 46, 53, 66, 75, 78–79
Cobalt salt, 31
Cochineal, 46
Coconut juice, 185
Cold, common, 111–112
Collagen, 107–108
Commoner, Dr. Barry, 22–23, 24
Constipation, 114–115, 184
Consumer Advisory Council, 167
Consumer Federation of America, 167
Consumerism, 165–168
Consumer legislation, 168
Consumer's Dictionary of Food Additives, A (Winter), 195
Consumers' Research, 166
Consumers Union of the United States, Inc., 166–167, 168
Control mechanisms of body, 134–135
Copper, 38, 43, 104
Copper sulfate, 42–43
Cosmetics, 71–79
Coumarin, 31
Crane, Dr. George W., 158
Cream, synthetic, 62
Cucumber juice, 183, 184–185
Cyclamates, 31, 67–70

Dandelion juice, 185
Darby, Dr. William J., 148, 149
Date juice, 186
DDT, 3–7, 11, 12, 13, 15, 22, 49, 152, 178
Deafness, 102–103
Deaths
due to heart trouble, 97, 117
as result of chemicals, 2, 10–11
Deficiency diseases, 97–117. See also Alcoholism, Mental illnesses
DeKruif, Dr. Paul, 116
Delaney, James J., 149
Dementia, 125
Demeton, 7, 10
Dentifrices, 75–77
Deodorants, 77–78
DES (diethylstilbestrol), 35, 40, 198–199
Detached retina, 101–102
Detergents in milk, 50
Dextrin, 198
Diacetyl, 65
Dieldrin, 7, 15
Diglycerides, 65, 200
Disodium guanylate, 199
Disodium phosphate, 52, 199
Drugs, 81–94
DuBois, Dr. Kenneth P., 11–12
Dulcin, 31
Dunbar, Paul, 37
Dunlop, Sir Derrick, 112
Durham, William F., 9

Economic action against body pollution, 169
EDTA (ethylinediamine tetraacetate), 199–200
Edwards, Charles C., 157
EFA (essential fatty acid), 64
Egler, Dr. Frank, 152
Emotional illnesses. See Mental illnesses
Emphysema, pulmonary, 113
Endocrine glands, 117

Environmental Defense Fund, 170
Enzymes, 29–30, 42, 48, 125
Epstein, Samuel S., 24
Estrin, 50
Estrogens, 73, 198
Ethylene glycol, 29
Exercise, amount of, in a reducing program, 119
Extenders, 47
Eye trouble, 98–99, 100–102

Farago, Dr. Peter, 86
Fasting, 173–179
Fat foods, how to eat, 193
FDA. See Food and Drug Administration
FD and C colors, 200
Federal Environment Pesticide Control Act, 15
Fennel juice, 185
Fertilizers, chemical, 17–26
farmers' dependence on, 18–19
harmful effects of, 22–25
proper use of, 20–21
Fine, Ralph Adam, 93
Fish, 47–49
Flavorings, 28, 36
Fleming, Dr., 141
Fluorides, 104–105
Follicular hyperkeratosis, 105
Food combining, 187–194
Food and Drug Administration, 4–5, 31–33, 54, 67–69
attempt of, to control sale of food supplements, 153–159
and news media, 159–161
and prescription drugs, 87–93
proper use of, 161–163
Food and Drug Law Institute (FDLI), 149–150
Food dyes, 35, 65
Food industry, 143–147
science research sponsored by, 147–149
Food and Nutrition Board, 154

Food Protection Committee, 67–68
Food wrappings and coatings, 35–36
Forman, Dr. Jonathan, 44
Freeman, Orville, 100
Freezing, 48
Freud, Sigmund, 121–122
Fruits, how to eat, 187–188
Functional properties, additives used to improve, 29
Fungicides, 2, 8

Garrison, Omar V., 158, 160
Genetotrophic individuality, 137–138
George, Dr. John L., 3, 7
Glucose. See Blood sugar
Glucose tolerance test, 127
Glutamine, 140
Glycerides, 200
Glycerine, 28
Glycogen, 123
Glycolysis, 125
Goddard, Dr. James L., 27–28, 154, 160
Goodman, Dr. Robert N., 9
Grapefruit juice, 181, 185, 186
GRAS (Generally Recognized As Safe) list, 69, 196
Gross, Dr. Jerome, 107
Gum arabic, 75

Hair, died and, 106
Hair dyes, 75
Hair-setting lotions, 74
Hair sprays, 75
Hamburgers, 45–46
Harvey, John L., 88
Heart disease, 109–110
Heinrichs, Dr. William L., 12
Herbicides, 2, 8
Heredity, alcoholism and, 137–138, 139
Hesperidin, 69
Heuper, Dr. W. C., 35–36, 54
Hexacholorophene, 77–78

High blood pressure. See Hypertension
Hog raising, 42–44
Honey, 56–57
Hormones, synthetic, 35, 42, 50
Hot dogs, 46–47
Howard, Sir Albert, 18
Hunter, Beatrice Trum, 149
Hydrochloric acid, 108
Hydrogenation, 63–65
Hydrogen peroxide, 49, 53
Hypertension, 87, 110–111
Hypothalamus, 138

Ice cream, 53–54
Ichthyosis, 88
Imitation flavor, 200–201
Infant formulas, 57–58
Infant mortality rates, 97
Infants
  DDT and, 5
  deaths of, 23–24
  food for, 57–59
Inorganic insecticides, 8
Inosinate, 201
Insecticides, 2–8
Iodine, 104
Iron, 104, 119, 182, 184
Isopropyl citrate, 65

Jordan, Carson, 88
Juices, raw, 180–186
Jukes, Dr. Thomas H., 155

Kelley, Dr. Gary, 22
Kelsey, Dr. Frances, 89–92, 162
Keratomalacia, 101
Kevadon (Thalidomide), 89–93, 150
Keys, Dr. Ancel, 64
King, Dr. Charles Glen, 148, 149
Kunde, Dr., 175

Larrick, George P., 31, 153–154
Laxatives, 84–85, 115
Lecithin, 65, 111, 201

Legal action against body pollution, 170–171
Lettuce juice, 184
Life expectancy of average American, 95–97
Linoleic acid, 111
Lipsticks, 78
Lithium chloride, 31
Liver, 123, 124
  diseases of the, 115–116
Longgood, William, 4–5, 9, 13, 143–144, 148
Lung cancer, 112
Lutz, Karl Barr, 107

McHenry, Dr. Eloise, 38
McHenry, Dr. Tom, 38
Mader, Dr. Donald Lewis, 22
Magnesium, 104, 108, 184
Malathion, 5
Maleic hydride, 29
Malnutrition of Americans, 98–100
Maple syrup, 56
Margarine, 63–64
Meat, ground, 45–47. See also Beef
Mellanby, Sir Edward, 38
Meniere's syndrome, 102–103
Mental illnesses, 121–129
Menthol, 201
Mercury, 49
Merrell Company, 87–93
MER/29, 87–89, 92–93, 150
Metabolic rate, 175
Methemoglobinemia, 23–24
Methenamine, 196
Methoxychlor, 5
Methyl bromide, 57
Milk, 49–53
  synthetic, 62–63
Minerals, 108, 109, 118, 119, 140, 183
Miticides, 2, 8, 14
Moisture controls, 28–29
Monoglycerides, 65, 200
Monsen, Dr. E. R., 62

Morey, Dr. Ray, 155
MSG (monosodium glutamate), 201–202
Mucilages, synthetic, 36

National Academy of Sciences' National Research Council (NAS-NRC), 151–152, 153, 154
Natural resistant crops, 14–15
NDGA (nordihydroguairetic acid), 32–33, 53
Nestor, Dr. John, 89
News media, 159–160
Niacin, 125
Nickel, 65
Nicotine, 14
Nitrates, 23–25, 202
Nitrites, 23–24, 202–203
Nitrous oxide, 57
Nutrition Foundation, Inc., 146–149
Nutrition and Your Mind: The Psychochemical Response (Watson), 127
Nutritional supplements, 29

O-acetate, 124, 125, 128
Obesity, 117–118
100,000,000 Guinea Pigs (Kallet and Schlink), 166
Onion and garlic juices, 185
Orange juice, 181, 185, 186
Organic farming, 18, 20, 25
Organic phosphates, 7, 8, 10, 12, 13
Osteoporosis, 108–109
Overeating, how to restrict, 118–119. See also Obesity
Overfed but Undernourished (Wood), 99
Oxidation of blood sugar, 124–125
Ozone, 49

Palopoli, Frank, 87
Pantothenic acid, 141
Papain, 42

Papaya juice, 114
Paradiaminobenzenes, 75
Paradichlorobenzene, 57
Paraffin, 36, 51
Paraformaldehyde, 56
Parathyroid glands, 135
Parsley juice, 182, 183
Parthion, 7, 10, 11
Pauling, Dr. Linus, 111
Pectin, 203
Pellagra, 105, 125
Penicillin, 50, 53
Perkin, William Henry, 66
Personal actions against body pollution, 173–186
Pesticides, 1, 2–15, 51
  and chemical fertilizers, 22
Phenol, 57
Phenylpropanolamine, 86
Phosdrin, 7, 10
Phosphoric acid, 29
Phosphorus, 98, 104, 108, 135, 183, 184
Physiologic activity agents, 29
Pineapple juice, 186
Poisons in Your Food, The (Longgood), 143–144, 148
Polycyclic aromatic compounds, 36
Polycyclic hydrocarbons, 55
Polyunsaturated fat, 63
Polyvinylpyrolidone, 75
Potassium citrate, 203
Potassium nitrate, 202
Potassium nitrite, 202
Pottinger, Dr. Francis M., Jr., 52
Poultry raising, 44–45
Prescription drugs, 86–94
Price, Dr. Weston A., 103–104
Processing aids, 28
Propionic anhydride, 57
Protein, 119, 123
  how to eat, 188, 192–194
  lack of, in American diet, 98
  in treating arthritis, 108
Prune juice, 186

Psychochemical cure for mental disorders, 126–129
Psychochemical states caused by nonfoods, 128–129
Ptyalin, 192
Pyorrhea, 184
Pyrethrum, 14
Pyruvate, 124, 125, 128

Radish juice, 183, 185–186
Raw juice therapy, 179–186
Red Dye No. 1, 31
Reid, Mary E., 107–108
Riboflavin, 181
Rice, Thomas, 88
Rosenthal, Benjamin S., 93
Rotenone, 14

Saccharin, 66–68
Safrole, 31
Salicylic acid (aspirin), 82
Salmonella bacteria, 41
Salt, in baby food, 58–59
Schizophrenia, 122–124, 126
Scientists, food industry and, 151–152
Sebrell, Dr. W. M., Jr., 154–155
Selikoff, Dr. Irving, 33
Shampoos, 74
Shaw, James H., 145
Shedan, Moses, 118
Shute, Dr. Wilfred E., 110
Sierra Club, 170
Silicon compounds, 35
Sinclair, Dr. Hugh, 108
Sinus cavities, cleansing of, 183
Skin
  cosmetics for, 72–73
  diseases of, 105
  functions of, 71–72
Smoking, 110, 111, 112–113
Social action against body pollution, 170
Sodium benzoate, 49, 65
Sodium bicarbonate, 76

Sodium bisulfite, 203
Sodium borate, 83
Sodium carrageenan, 197
Sodium citrate, 52, 203
Sodium nicotinate, 46
Sodium nitrate, 196, 202
Sodium nitrite, 28, 46, 49, 202
Sodium salicylate, 82, 196
Sodium sulfite, 46
Soil, 17
    loss of, 18–20, 25
    sponge structure of, 21
Sorbitol, 203–204
Spinach juice, 184, 185
Stabilizers, 53
Staphylococci, 53
Starch, how to eat, 188, 192, 194
Stare, Dr. Frederick J., 141, 147–
    148, 156–157
Starkey, Mrs. Ione Dennis, 27
Stearyl citrate, 65
Stewart, Dr. William, 156
Strawberry juice, 186
Streptococci, 53
Strontium-90, 51
Sugar, 54–57, 145–146
    how to eat, 194
    synthetic substitutes for, 66–70
Sugar Research Foundation, 145–
    146
Sulfur, 183, 184
Supermarket Institute, 144
Surfactants, 36
Sweeteners, artificial, 66–70
Synergists, 8, 33
Synthetic foodstuffs, 61–65
Systemic insecticides, 8

Tenderizers, 42, 44, 47
TEPP (tetraethyl pyrophosphate), 7,
    11
Thalidomide, 89–93, 162
Theobromine sodium salicylate, 196
Thioglycerides, 74
Thyroid gland, 117, 122

Tinnitus, 102
Tolerance levels of chemicals, 5
Tomato juice, 185
Tooth decay, 76, 98, 103–105, 176
Toothpaste, 75–77
Trace elements, 21
Tranquilizers, 40–41, 44, 50
Trulson, Dr., 141
Turnip leaf juice, 184

Ulcers, stomach, 113–114
UN Joint FAO/WHO, 32, 59
United States
    health in, 95–120
    life expectancy in, 95–97
    malnutrition in, 98–100
United States Government
    food additives and, 30–33, 149
    food industry and, 149–152
    See also Food and Drug Adminis-
        tration
Unsaturated fats, 108

Vitamin A, 99, 100–101, 102, 104,
    105, 182
Vitamin B complex, 98, 102, 105,
    106, 111, 116, 119, 182
Vitamin C, 100, 102, 104, 107, 110,
    111–112, 114, 155, 181, 186,
    196
Vitamin D, 52, 109
Vitamin E, 110, 111, 119, 182
Vitamin K, 181, 182
Vitamins
    effect of chemical additives on,
        29–30
    lack of, in American diets, 98
    supplements used to treat alcohol-
        ism, 139–140, 141
    synthetic, 65
Vitamins in Medicine, The (Bicknell
    and Prescott), 107
VonLiebig, Justus, 17
Voris, Dr. LeRoy, 154

Walsh, Dr. Michael, H., 55
Watercress juice, 184
Watson, Dr. George, 122, 126, 146
Weider, Dr. Steve, 155
Weight reducing drugs, 85–86
Weissenberg, Sidney, 156
Wheat germ, 37, 119
Wickenden, Leonard, 151
Williams, Dr. Roger J., 132, 133, 134, 139, 140–141, 142

Winter, Ruth, 195
Wolfe, Homer R., 9
Wood, Dr. H. Curtis, Jr., 99, 100, 111

Xerothalmia, 100

Young, James Harvey, 160
Yudkin, Dr. John, 55–56, 146